Case-Based Inpatient Pediatric Dermatology

Marcia Hogeling

Editor

Case-Based Inpatient Pediatric Dermatology

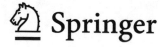 Springer

Editor
Marcia Hogeling
Director of Pediatric Dermatology
UCLA Division of Dermatology
Los Angeles, CA, USA

ISBN 978-3-319-81066-9   ISBN 978-3-319-31569-0   (eBook)
DOI 10.1007/978-3-319-31569-0

Printed on acid-free paper

This Springer imprint is published by Springer Nature
The registered company is Springer International Publishing AG Switzerland

For Yaron

Preface

Case-based inpatient pediatric dermatology is an approach to pediatric skin disease specific to hospitalized children. The idea for the book initially came from doing a talk on interesting inpatient dermatology cases and realizing there was no specific resource book for this niche of pediatric dermatology.

Skin problems make up to one third of patient complaints, and although dermatology is primarily an outpatient specialty, there are specific cutaneous diseases that are more commonly seen in hospitalized children.

The book is geared as a reference toward a diverse audience including hospitalists, emergency and inpatient clinicians, pediatricians, dermatologists, residents, and medical students.

The book is organized into a question-and-answer format that should make it more interactive and helpful for those that are studying for exams and to learn specific teaching pearls.

There are 14 chapters with associated images to provide you clinical examples.

To make this book possible, I have been blessed by the help from many brilliant and generous colleagues from across the country and overseas, who have contributed their time and expertise to writing chapters. I thank them for their great efforts in creating this book. Thanks to Connie Walsh, developmental editor, for her invaluable assistance. I also thank my mentors, who have taught me academic pediatric dermatology, and my patients, who are a daily inspiration.

I hope that you will find this book to be a valuable resource and guide.

Los Angeles, CA, USA   Marcia Hogeling

Contents

Contributors

Luluah Al-Mubarak, MD Department of Dermatology, Prince Sultan Military Medical City, Riyadh, Saudi Arabia

Sarah Asch, MD Department of Dermatology, Mayo Clinic, Rochester, MN, USA

Adam Bartlett, BSc, MBBS, MPHTM Department of Immunology and Infectious Diseases, Sydney Children's Hospital, Randwick, NSW, Australia

Christina L. Boull, MD Department of Pediatric Dermatology, University of Minnesota, Minneapolis, MN, USA

Heather A. Brandling-Bennett, MD Division of Dermatology, Department of Pediatrics, Seattle Children's Hospital/University of Washington, Seattle, WA, USA

Colleen Cotton, MD Division of Dermatology, Department of Medicine, University of Arizona, Tucson, AZ, USA

Sheila Fallon Friedlander, MD Department of Dermatology and Pediatrics, University of California San Diego School of Medicine/Rady Children's Hospital, San Diego, CA, USA

Ellen S. Haddock, MBA. Department of Pediatric and Adolescent Dermatology, University of California, San Diego, CA, USA

Nicole N. Harter, BS, MD Department of Dermatology, Children's Hospital Los Angeles, Keck School of Medicine of USC, Los Angeles, CA, USA

Marcia Hogeling, MD Division of Dermatology, University of California, Los Angeles, Los Angeles, CA, USA

Jennifer T. Huang, MD Dermatology Program, Boston Children's Hospital, Harvard Medical School, Boston, MA, USA

Kimberly Jablon, MD Department of Pediatrics, UCSF Benioff Childrens' Hospital, San Francisco, CA, USA

Hasan Khosravi, BS Harvard Medical School, Boston, MA, USA

Minnelly Luu, MD Department of Dermatology, Children's Hospital Los Angeles, Keck School of Medicine of USC, Los Angeles, CA, USA

Sheilagh M. Maguiness, MD Department of Pediatric Dermatology, University of Minnesota, Minneapolis, MN, USA

Erin Mathes, MD Department of Dermatology and Pediatrics, University of California, San Francisco, San Francisco, CA, USA

Catalina Matiz, MD Division of Pediatric and Adolescent Dermatology, University of California, San Diego, CA, USA

Division of Pediatric and Adolescent Dermatology, Department of Dermatology, Rady Children's Hospital, San Diego, CA, USA

Patrick McMahon, MD Department of Pediatric Dermatology, The Children's Hospital of Philadelphia, Philadelphia, PA, USA

The Perelman School of Medicine at the University of Pennsylvania, Philadelphia, PA, USA

Anar Mikailov, MD Harvard Combined Medicine-Dermatology Residency Program, Boston, MA, USA

Kimberly D. Morel, MD, FAAD, FAAP Department of Dermatology and Pediatrics, Morgan Stanley Children's Hospital of New York-Presbyterian/Columbia University, New York, NY, USA

Emily Osier, MD Division of Pediatric and Adolescent Dermatology, Department of Dermatology, University of California, San Diego, CA, USA

Division of Pediatric and Adolescent Dermatology, Department of Dermatology, Rady Children's Hospital, San Diego, CA, USA

Pamela Palasanthiran, MBBS, MD, FRACP Department of Immunology and Infectious Diseases, Sydney Children's Hospital, Randwick, NSW, Australia

Kara N. Shah, MD, PhD Division of Dermatology, Cincinnati Children's Hospital, Cincinnati, OH, USA

Kirsten Simonton, MD Mayerson Center for Safe and Healthy Children, Cincinnati Children's Hospital, Cincinnati, OH, USA

Robert James Smith, BS Department of Pediatric Dermatology, The Children's Hospital of Philadelphia, Philadelphia, PA, USA

The Perelman School of Medicine at the University of Pennsylvania, Philadelphia, PA, USA

Clayton Sontheimer, MD Division of Rheumatology, Department of Pediatrics, Seattle Children's Hospital/University of Washington, Seattle, WA, USA

Marion E. Tamesis, MD Department of Dermatology, New York Presbyterian Hospital, Columbia University Medical Center, New York, NY, USA

Megha M. Tollefson, MD Department of Dermatology and Pediatrics, Mayo Clinic, Rochester, MN, USA

Wynnis L. Tom, MD Department of Dermatology and Pediatrics, University of California, San Diego and Rady Children's Hospital, San Diego, CA, USA

Orli Wargon, MBBS (Hons1), MClinEd, FACD Department Pediatric Dermatology, Sydney Children's Hospital, Randwick, NSW, Australia

Chapter 1
Atopic Dermatitis and Papulosquamous Disorders

Sarah Asch and Megha M. Tollefson

Abstract It is not uncommon to encounter certain papulosquamous diseases in an inpatient setting in general pediatrics. At times, the skin disease is the primary reason for admission; while in others, recognition of the skin disease may be relevant to ongoing care, such as continued appropriate topical therapy for a patient's atopic dermatitis. Skin disease is not an uncommon reason for admission, and patients occasionally acquire a skin problem in the hospital, such as severe diaper dermatitis. Recognition of dermatologic diseases early on may shorten hospitalizations over all, and should lead to better management with appropriate consult and coordination of care.

Keywords Psoriasis • Atopic dermatitis • Diaper dermatitis • Allergic contact dermatitis • Wiskott–Aldrich • Omenn

Case 1.1. Atopic Dermatitis

A 4-year-old child with a known history of moderate atopic dermatitis, allergic rhinitis, and mild asthma returns from weeklong camping trip to the Arizona desert in February. During vacation, family was unable to apply moisturizer daily, but did apply 1 % hydrocortisone as recommended on most days. Patient took only one shower during the trip and no baths. The patient did not swim while away. Patient's atopic dermatitis flared slightly while on trip, but a few days after return the flare continued and is now out of control 2 weeks later.

She saw her PCP who prescribed a course of oral antibiotics for impetiginized areas, but patient has only improved slightly. Patient currently waking each night to scratch, finding blood on sheets in the morning; weeping patches at ankles,

S. Asch, MD
Department of Dermatology, Mayo Clinic, Rochester, MN, USA
e-mail: asch.sarah@mayo.edu

M.M. Tollefson, MD (✉)
Departments of Dermatology and Pediatrics, Mayo Clinic, Rochester, MN, USA
e-mail: Tollefson.megha@mayo.edu

© Springer International Publishing Switzerland 2016
M. Hogeling (ed.), *Case-Based Inpatient Pediatric Dermatology*,
DOI 10.1007/978-3-319-31569-0_1

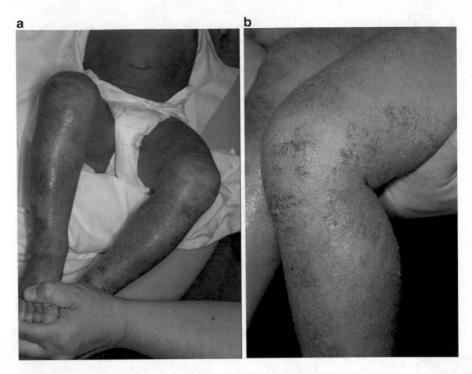

Fig. 1.1 (a), (b). A 4-year-old child with flare of moderate atopic dermatitis

wrists, as well as popliteal fossae and antecubital fossae are persistent and unresponsive to topical steroids and ointment moisturizer. Patient is co-sleeping due to all the discomfort and unable to go to daycare due to itching and the weeping plaques (Fig. 1.1).

Labs

Cultures of skin have shown Methicillin-sensitive Staphylococcus Aureus in the past.

Questions

1. What, if any, further workup would you perform?
2. What systemic treatments would you employ for this patient?
3. What is the role for topical treatment in patients with this severity of atopic dermatitis flare?

Discussion

Atopic dermatitis (AD) is a common chronic inflammatory condition that affects all age groups and disproportionately affects the pediatric population. AD is an issue of paramount importance to clinical practice of pediatricians and dermatologists alike. Pediatric atopic dermatitis can disrupt normal growth and development of affected children, lead to secondary infection, significantly affect the quality of life of families with affected children, and be financially burdensome [1, 2]. The importance of evidence-based treatment guidelines for this chronic illness was highlighted by the publication in 2014–2015 of a 4 part series in the Journal of the American Academy of Dermatology entitled: Guidelines of care for the management of atopic dermatitis. A summary and review with practical tips for primary care pediatricians including a succinct treatment algorithm was published in Pediatrics in 2015 [3].

Treatment of all pediatric atopic dermatitis has five components that must all be addressed simultaneously in order to heal the skin and prevent flares.

1. Repair the skin barrier
2. Treat inflammation
3. Treat superinfections
4. Identify and remove triggers
5. Educate the patient and caregivers about the nature of this chronic remitting and relapsing disease

Roles of Topical Treatments: Barrier Repair and Inflammation

Barrier repair is the cornerstone of atopic dermatitis care. When patients leave the hospital, it is critical that they have the tools and understand the importance of maintaining the barrier. In the hospital, this can be well accomplished with moisturizing the skin. In general in dermatology practice, ointments (clear, greasy substances such as white petrolatum) are preferred for sealing moisture into skin. The soak and smear method is commonly employed in outpatient dermatology and can be translated to the hospital setting. The basics are a soak for 10–15 min in a comfortable temperature bathtub, then to apply the medicated ointments and then a layer of emollient. The absorption can be increased with occlusion and often putting damp dressings (or pajamas) over the ointments, followed by warm blankets to keep the patient comfortable. At Mayo Clinic, wet dressings have been used for many years for inpatient atopic dermatitis (Fig. 1.2) and involve applying medicated creams (white substances) and then applying wet to dry dressings, to which dilute acetic acid may be added to help treat superinfections. This is repeated every 3–4 h, and can include treatment to the face as well [4].

Inflammation is a driving force in atopic dermatitis, and providing adequate treatment especially through skin-directed therapy can be challenging at all ages. When patients are hospitalized, demonstrating that skin-directed therapy is safe and effective is important for outpatient success. Topical steroids are the mainstay of treatment of inflammation in atopic dermatitis. In the hospitalized patient, one com-

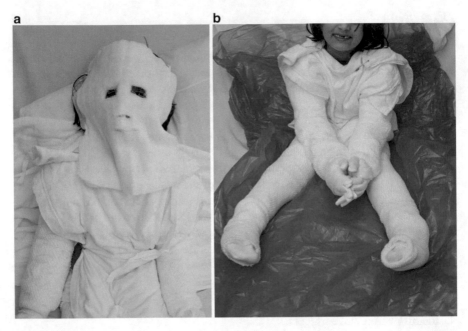

Fig. 1.2 (**a**), (**b**). A 6-year-old child with atopic dermatitis in wet dressings

mon challenge is obtaining sufficient quantities for application due to miscommunications between physicians and bedside staff or the pharmacy. The physician must pay close attention to the quantities ordered to ensure sufficient amounts are delivered to the bedside. A helpful trick can be to order a 1-lb (454 g) jar to the bedside for the body application; this should be enough to treat an adult body surface area twice daily for 1 week. In children and infants, these quantities are less (~250 g for a child, ~100 g for an infant) [3]; however, medications in larger jars are often easier to apply than those in smaller tubes. Medicated ointments or creams should be applied prior to moisturizers to help increase penetration into the skin. The medications are generally felt to be absorbed within 30 min.

Roles for Systemic Therapies: Pruritus and Infection

A second key part to barrier repair is to prevent scratching or rubbing, thus bringing mechanical damage to the barrier. The most effective way to do this is to repair the barrier, which improves itch dramatically. Itch is often the most difficult symptom to treat. Use of sedating antihistamines at bedtime to prevent overnight scratching is utilized during acute flares; while these medications do not effectively treat the itch, they are useful in assisting in undisturbed sleep. Daytime non-sedating or lower dose sedating antihistamines are not recommended because they are less effective than direct barrier repair and treatment of the inflammation as the itch is not directly histamine driven [5]. If the skin is not markedly improved after aggressive topical therapy for 48 h, oral antibiotics may also be added depending on culture results (see below).

Role of Infection and Further Workup: Surveillance Cultures

In the pediatric patient who has been hospitalized for their atopic dermatitis, infection is a common reason for flare. Infection is most commonly from S. Aureus (MSSA or MRSA), but viral superinfection with HSV (eczema herpeticum) or coxsackie (eczema coxsackium) can also lead to flares. In contrast to the usual teaching in pediatrics, dermatologists will frequently swab areas that do not appear overtly impetiginized for surveillance cultures. This allows therapy to be tailored more accurately if the patient is not improving with barrier repair and treatment of inflammation. Skin infection in atopic patients may require primary treatment with oral antibiotics, specifically an antibiotic that has adequate coverage of Gram-positive bacteria. Should the patient have a history of MRSA, cultures of the skin should be taken and used to tailor therapy. If needed, coverage for MRSA can be utilized; however, it is important to remember that while TMP-Sulfa methoxazole is often used for MRSA, it has less adequate Streptococcal coverage and thus is not generally used first line in these patients.

Bleach baths have become widely used and are now the standard of care in the management of atopic dermatitis. However, even in the best-collected clinical evidence evaluated by a panel of experts in dermatology, evidence-based guidelines for bathing were still difficult to establish. At this time, we recommend approximately ½ cup of regular household bleach to a full bathtub (approximately 40 gal) of water. Regular household bleach has recently increased in concentration from 6 to 8.25 %, and thus some experts now recommend only about 1/3 cup of bleach to a full bathtub. One must caution parents to never apply bleach directly to the child's skin, as this can cause a chemical burn [6].

Identification of triggers can be challenging and is often best addressed on an outpatient basis. Common triggers include change of seasons, new more humid or drier environment, stress, airborne allergens, fragrances, and skin infections. Food allergy requires special comment, as parents often remove whole classes of foods to attempt to control atopic dermatitis, and strict elimination diets without proper nutritional guidance can lead to poor growth due to inadequate nutrition. In general, atopic dermatitis is rarely directly related to food allergy [7]. An expert panel sponsored by the NIAID (National Institute of Allergy and Infectious Diseases; a branch of the National Institutes of Health (NIH)) recommends testing for milk, egg, peanut, wheat, and soy in children under 5 years of age with moderate to severe atopic dermatitis, only if the child has persistent AD *in spite of optimized management* and topical therapy; or if the patient has a reliable history of an immediate reaction after ingestion of a specific food. The expert panel specifically recommends against avoiding *potential* allergenic foods as a means of controlling atopic dermatitis [8]. Should food allergy be a consideration for exacerbation of an individual's atopic dermatitis, we recommend referral to an allergist for appropriate testing to determine if true food allergies are present, so that the child's diet is not unnecessarily restricted.

Education of caregivers and the patient is critical to control of atopic dermatitis. Daily ongoing moisturization of the barrier is key for many patients, and adjusting this with age-appropriate considerations is important [3]. For example, a 4-year-old is often more likely to tolerate an ointment preparation than an adolescent. However, each person is truly individual and it is most helpful to ask, as a tube of medicine kept in a drawer (and hence not applied to the skin) is not effective for any skin disease.

There are times when oral immunosuppressive drugs are required to manage chronic uncontrolled atopic dermatitis. However, the vast majority of patients can be managed with aggressive topical treatments as outlined above.

Answers

1. Surveillance cultures.
2. Sedating antihistamines. If skin not markedly improved in 2 days, then oral antibiotics based on culture results and clinical exam.
3. Topical treatments with goal of barrier repair and decreasing inflammation are the mainstay of therapy. Wet dressings can be helpful adjunct both inpatient and modified therapy as outpatient.

Case 1.2. Pustular Psoriasis

A 2-year-old girl presents with acute onset of a widespread pustular eruption after recovering from a viral illness. She has been using topical creams at home for the last week, without improvement. She has been treated for cradle cap and intertrigo intermittently since 5 months of age. At age one, she had hand-foot-and-mouth disease, after which she developed a pustular eruption similar to the current findings, but with more limited involvement. She had a biopsy at that time consistent with pustular psoriasis.

Physical Exam

- T 38.5 °C, vital signs otherwise within normal limits for age
- General: tired, but nontoxic appearing child, seated on mom's lap
- Skin exam elicits some tenderness of her skin. She has a widespread erythematous eruption consisting of sharply demarcated pink-red thin plaques. Some of the plaques are studded with tiny pustules. Her finger and toenails are not involved. She has geographic tongue (Fig. 1.3)

Labs

CBC with differential, electrolytes including calcium, and liver function tests are within normal range.

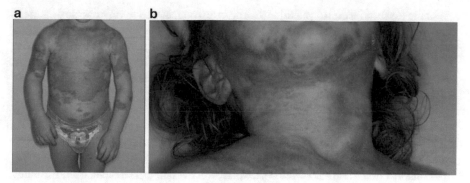

Fig. 1.3 (a), (b). A 2-year-old child with pustular psoriasis

Questions

1. What is the role of systemic steroids in psoriasis?
2. What laboratory value should be closely monitored in patients with pustular psoriasis flares?

Discussion

Pustular psoriasis is an uncommon but severe form of psoriasis, often requiring hospitalization and systemic treatment. It can often be complicated by cutaneous infection or even sepsis. A second severe form of psoriasis is erythrodermic or exfoliative psoriasis. Together these two forms occur in about 1 % of pediatric psoriasis patients [9]. Patients with either of these presentations may have failure to thrive due to excessive energies spent on their skin disease. As opposed to adults, who often carry a preexisting diagnosis of psoriasis, infants and children can present with pustular psoriasis as their initial episode of skin disease—as early as 1 week of life. Pustular psoriasis commonly recurs with increasing severity and accordingly, worsening prognosis. However, the disease can remain quiescent for decades, only to recur unexpectedly without identifiable trigger. The cause of pustular psoriasis in children is unknown, although there is likely a genetic basis [9].

Pustular psoriasis is usually generalized and presents with sudden onset of fever, malaise, and anorexia. The accompanying skin rapidly develops superficial 1–3 mm pustules, often overlying erythematous annular plaques or patches. The pustules can coalesce and form sheets or lakes of pus, especially in flexures, genitals, interdigital spaces, and periungually. Nails are often affected and can become thickened or separate from the nail bed with pus. Oral lesions including the tongue are not uncommon and resemble geographic tongue [10]. As the inflammation resolves, the pustules crust and affected skin will slough.

Acute erythrodermic or pustular psoriasis are considered dermatologic emergencies and require hospitalization for treatment. Skin biopsy and laboratory testing can be helpful in distinguishing this from other causes of widespread pustules. The differential diagnosis includes cutaneous Candidiasis, Staphylococcal infection, Herpes simplex, Acute Generalized Exanthematous Pustulosis (AGEP), Eosinophilic folliculitis, and Deficiency of Interleukin 1 Receptor antagonist (DIRA).

Management often includes supportive care, sometimes in an ICU setting, as well as skin-directed and systemic therapies. Hypocalcemia can occur and calcium should be monitored. If topical treatments with corticosteroids and wet dressings or compresses fail, systemic therapy is warranted.

Similar to treatment for atopic dermatitis, wet dressings have been used for many years at Mayo Clinic. This skin-directed treatment involves applying medicated creams (white substances) such as topical triamcinolone, and then applying wet to dry dressings, to which dilute acetic acid may be added to help treat superinfections. This is repeated every 3–4 h and can include treatment to the face as well [4]. This requires significant nursing care, and thus sometimes patients can be more easily treated in an ICU setting in some institutions where nurse to patient ratios are lower. This is particularly appropriate for patients with pustular psoriasis who can be quite ill at baseline and warrant close monitoring.

Dermatologists warn strongly against use of systemic corticosteroids in treatment of plaque psoriasis due to significant rebound flares or even inducing pustular psoriasis; however, in ICU and other settings where the child is quite ill, occasionally corticosteroids are very judiciously used while initiating other therapies. Acitretin and isotretinoin are oral retinoids (Vitamin A derivatives), which have been used as first-line therapy for pustular psoriasis. Cyclosporine is another commonly used systemic agent in pustular psoriasis, due to its high rate of efficacy and quick onset of action. Methotrexate is sometimes utilized in this setting, but has slower onset of action; thus, it is often used in conjunction with an agent that has a more rapid onset of action. Biologic therapies are now increasingly becoming first-line therapy for severe and recurrent cases, but onset of action is also slower, and evaluation for latent infections including TB and Hepatitis must be completed prior to initiation of therapy [9, 10].

Another treatment that is extremely effective, but is not widely available, is Goeckerman therapy. This employs daily phototherapy followed by application of crude coal tar mixtures to the entire body including the scalp. Patients are then wrapped in plastic and shower caps, followed by pajamas or scrubs. While very effective, it is only performed at a few locations around the country, including Mayo Clinic, University of California, San Francisco and University of Michigan. It has fallen out of favor due to the labor-intensive nature of the therapy, for both patient and provider; however, it remains an excellent therapy for psoriasis and induces long remissions in most patients without the need for systemic treatment [11].

Answers

1. Generally, we discourage use of systemic steroids in psoriasis, due to risk for rebound flare, with pustular psoriasis as the most notable exception to this rule of thumb.
2. Calcium is the most well known associated derangement. Patients should also be monitored for electrolyte imbalances and adequate hydration in keeping with standard supportive measures in very ill patients.

Case 1.3. Allergic or Irritant Contact Dermatitis

A 6-year-old male has had molluscum for several months. He has been treated with topical imiquimod without effect, thus this was discontinued 2 months ago. Mom noted new spots behind his left ear and on his neck a few days prior to admission. She applied topical Neosporin, as she would do for any skin breakage, at least twice daily for 2 days. The patient then developed erythema, erosion, and edema in the areas where the Neosporin was used (Fig. 1.4).

Fig. 1.4 A 6-year old
male with allergic contact
dermatitis to neomycin

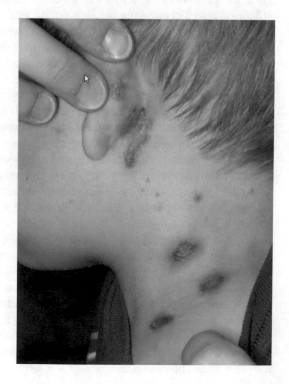

Labs

Culture of vesicles is negative for bacteria and herpes simplex virus.

Questions

1. What are three common causes of contact dermatitis in hospitalized patients?
2. What is the timing and natural history of allergic contact dermatitis?

Discussion

Contact dermatitis is an umbrella term that refers to dermatitis after coming into contact with a chemical agent. Both irritant and allergic contact dermatitis are seen in the inpatient setting. There are distinguishing features that are helpful clues in making a correct diagnosis. Irritant dermatitis is much more common, is often the basis of diaper dermatitis, and can also be from irritation from adhesive tape, or antiseptics used for procedures, such as chlorhexidine. Allergic contact dermatitis is much less common, especially in the inpatient setting. Allergic contact dermatitis is a delayed-type IV hypersensitivity reaction that requires sensitization (meaning exposure to the allergen prior to the current exposure). Delayed-type hypersensitivity sensitization can take days to years to develop and may happen suddenly despite years of exposures. But after sensitization, reexposure leads quickly to a rash often characterized by itching/pain, weeping rash, or even blisters in some cases [12].

Neomycin is a common allergic contact allergen, well known to dermatologists, and was the 2010 Contact Allergen of the year. It has been implicated in numerous studies of both pediatric and adult patients of contact dermatitis [13]. Many patients have already been sensitized to neomycin after use on cuts and scrapes in the USA and thus, a reaction within 1–2 days of reexposure is not unexpected. Of note, patients with neomycin allergy may also have co-sensitivity to bacitracin (likely due to similar exposure patterns). Also relevant to inpatient medicine, neomycin is an aminoglycoside and can cross-react with medicines in the same class including gentamicin and tobramycin.

Patterns in contact allergy change with time and exposures at the population level, thus research into an updated list of contact allergens can be helpful when evaluating a patient with a known exposure [14]. There a several resources for contact allergen information, including the American Contact Dermatitis Society and the North American Contact Dermatitis Group Patch test results are published regularly [15]. Several groups have conducted studies to assess for prevalence of various contact allergens; the most recent lists of pediatric contact allergens contain nickel, fragrance mix, neomycin, and formaldehyde. Other common offenders in pediatrics include cocamidopropyl betaine (used as a surfactant for "no tear" formulations and other foaming cleansers), Balsam of Peru, and methylisothiazolinone (found in many baby wipes) [16].

Chlorhexidine is an emerging contact allergen in the hospital. Chlorhexidine baths for all ICU patients is becoming the standard of care in some intensive care units both in adult and pediatric hospitals to lower central line infections and bacteremia [17, 18]. While data is still out on whether this is a truly effective intervention [19], there may be an increased risk for irritant or allergic contact dermatitis. Another common cause of irritant contact is from iodine (Betadine) that does not get completely washed from the skin after a surgical procedure [20]. It often underlies the edges of drapes and can take on a variety of geometric patterns. A thorough history regarding specifics of patient positioning during procedures can be extremely helpful in elucidating this diagnosis.

Answers

1. Chlorhexidine, Betadine, and tape
2. Slow onset after initial exposure (10 days–2 weeks), subsequent exposures are much faster with rash within 1–2 days

Case 1.4. Eczematous Eruptions as Sign of Underlying Disease

You are consulted to evaluate a 2-month-old male, admitted with fever, decreased urine output, tachycardia, and purulent umbilical drainage. Blood cultures grew *Enterococcus faecalis* and *Staphylococcus aureus*. The patient was born at full term with unremarkable birth history and good prenatal care. Prior to admission, his primary care physician diagnosed eczema due to a red scaly rash, and his formula was changed several times, due to concern for milk allergy.

On exam, he is an unwell, small appearing infant with red skin and slight scale from scalp to feet, somewhat sparing the diaper area. Scalp has significant yellow scale. No blisters or erosions are noted. Hepatosplenomegaly is noted on palpation of his abdomen (Fig. 1.5).

Labs

- White blood cell count 49 (6–14 K/μL)
- Eosinophils: 10.8 (0.1–1.6 K/μL)
- IgE: 2339 (<17 K/μL)
- IgG, IgM, IgA: low
- TRECS (T-cell receptor excision circles): absent

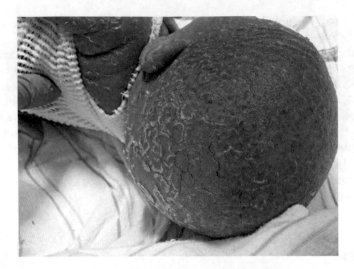

Fig. 1.5 Infant with eczematous eruption due to underlying immunodeficiency

Questions

1. What are genetic syndromes or disorders in the differential diagnosis for eczematous rash in infants? What is the diagnosis for this case?
2. What laboratory evaluations should you initially review or recommend to clarify the diagnosis?

Discussion

Individually, the underlying genetic disorders that lead to eczematous eruptions are rare. However, pediatricians may face these challenging diagnoses at some point in their careers. Wiskott–Aldrich syndrome, Hyper IgE Syndrome (HIES), Omenn syndrome, DiGeorge syndrome, Netherton's syndrome, selective IgA deficiency, and metabolic disorders such as phenylketonuria can all present with eczematous eruptions. Table 1.1 helps to differentiate some of these diseases by the accompanying findings of each disorder [9, 21]. Final diagnosis will involve not only dermatology but may also require input from Immunology, Genetics, and/or Hematology colleagues [22].

A specific type of seborrheic dermatitis with severe generalized erythema and scale (called Leiner's phenotype) should trigger an evaluation for underlying immune deficiency. This was once thought to be a separate disease, but is now known to be a presenting sign of complement deficiencies, HIES, SCID (especially Omenn syndrome) and X-linked agammaglobulinemia [9]. In this patient, the laboratory values of eosinophilia, elevated IgE and absence of T cell excision circles

Table 1.1 Differentiating features of selected genetic disorders with eczematous rash

Disease	Differentiating cutaneous PE	Differentiating systems	Infections	Differentiating labs
Wiskott–Aldrich	Purpuric lesions, including mucocutaneous; cutaneous vasculitis	Bloody diarrhea, epistaxis, hepatosplenomegaly, arthritis	Recurrent bacterial: pneumococcus, H. influenzae, N. meningitides, herpes, and PJP	Thrombocytopenia
HIES	Facial/intertriginous Staph abscesses	Coarse facies, dental (retained primary teeth), bone (scoliosis)	Sinopulmonary infections; cutaneous candidiasis	Elevated IgE, eosinophilia
Omenn	"Leiner's phenotype" seborrheic dermatitis; extensive involvement	Hepatosplenomegaly (88 %) lymphadenopathy (80 %), alopecia (57 %); diarrhea, FTT	Candidal and pneumonia	Eosinophilia, elevated IgE

HIES Hyper IgE Syndrome, *H. influenzae* Haemophilus influenzae, *N. meningitides* Neisseria meningitides, *PJP* pneumocystis jiroveci pneumonia (formerly *PCP* Pneumocystis carinii pneumonia), *FTT* failure to thrive

(TRECS) suggested a diagnosis of Omenn syndrome, which is a type of severe combined immunodeficiency (SCID). A gene panel for SCID was ordered, and a mutation in Rag 2 was identified, confirming the diagnosis of Omenn syndrome. The patient was treated with wet wraps with topical triamcinolone and petrolatum initially, and then received an unrelated donor hematopoietic stem cell transplant, with significant improvement in his rash post-transplant.

Treatment of the underlying immunodeficiency with transplant can be helpful in some cases. One pitfall is that eczematous reactions can look very similar on skin biopsy to grade 1–2 graft versus host disease (GVHD) [23]. As children with some of these disorders are treated with bone marrow transplantation, it can be difficult to assess if the eruption is due to their underlying disease or harbingers onset of GVHD. The timing of rash with relation to transplant and changes in immunosuppressive medications, as well as distribution of the affected areas can sometimes be helpful in differentiating, but is not always possible.

Treatment of eczematous eruptions associated with underlying immunodeficiency follows the same principles as those of "garden variety" atopic dermatitis with skin-directed treatment including topical corticosteroids and sedating antihistamines at night, as well as a regimen of moisturizers and bathing (see Atopic Dermatitis case for more discussion of treatment). However, treatment of the skin disease associated with these conditions should not be taken lightly, as impaired barriers leave these patients at risk for infection and increased metabolic demands from the skin can impair growth.

Answers

1. Wiskott–Aldrich syndrome, Omenn syndrome, HIES (Hyper IgE syndrome), DiGeorge syndrome, Netherton's syndrome, selective IgA deficiency, and metabolic disorders such as phenylketonuria. The diagnosis for this case is Omenn syndrome.
2. CBC with differential for thrombocytopenia and eosinophilia; Total IgE. TRECS (T cell receptor excision circles—screen for severe combined immunodeficiency) are part of some state routine newborn screens. If considering this diagnosis, it is important to verify what your state newborn screen includes, as newborn screening is not nationally standardized.

Case 1.5. Severe Diaper Dermatitis

A 6-month-old infant girl with chronic diarrhea is undergoing evaluation for causes of her chronic diarrhea as an inpatient. She also requires management of the following diaper dermatitis. Parents have tried several different diaper creams, triple antibiotic ointment and have been using baby wipes and scrubbing down to clean skin between every change (Fig. 1.6).

Fig. 1.6 A 6-month-old
infant with pustules and
erythema in the diaper area

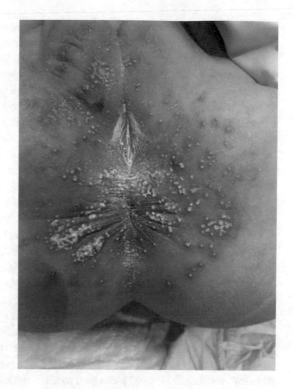

Labs

- Swab of the pustules is positive for Candida Albicans.

Questions

1. Name two systemic conditions that commonly involve the diaper area.
2. What is a key initial step in treating any diaper dermatitis?

Discussion

Treatment of significant diaper dermatitis can be very challenging. Severe diaper dermatitis goes by several different names, all largely felt to be on a spectrum of disease. Erosive diaper dermatitis, Pseudoverrucous papules and nodules, Granuloma gluteal infantum, and Jacquet's erosive diaper dermatitis all have similar presumed etiology [9, 21].

Most diaper dermatitis is multifactorial; it is often a compound problem of barrier breakdown, low-grade superinfection, the immature nature of newborn skin, and a difficult wound healing environment [24]. Irritants in diaper dermatitis usually affect the convex surfaces and relatively spare the folds, thus distinguishing irritant diaper dermatitis from other causes of diaper dermatitis. The barrier in the diaper area is constantly exposed to irritants from urine and stool, and these are often kept under occlusion (diapers), further irritating the area. Bile acids in acute diarrheal illness or chronic diarrhea are a significant irritant. Topical cholestyramine added to an ointment or zinc oxide base can bind bile acids and lessen the irritant potential from this component [25]. Contact dermatitis is another known cause of diaper dermatitis. Baby wipes with high levels of methylisothiazolinone have been implicated in some cases of diaper dermatitis, as well as the blue dye from diapers (more commonly seen along back at waistline). Another common contact allergen is neomycin, which is found in triple antibiotic ointments and while not frequently used in the diaper area, should always be on your list of questions, especially when parents may have been treating for a suspected infection.

Gentle skin care in the treatment of diaper dermatitis is of paramount importance. A key point to educate families and caregivers is that barrier creams must be put on very thickly (like cream cheese or frosting) and should not be completely removed with diaper changes, as this level of friction and scrubbing can irritate the skin. To remove these creams, mineral oil can be used to emulsify cream and wipe off gently, which allows for removal with less traumatic irritation to the area. When possible, leaving the diaper area open to air is desirable, but this is often impractical with children of diaper-wearing age or special needs. Thus, we often recommend dry diaper area thoroughly with air, by waving of hand or use of small handheld fan, and then replacing ointments or creams.

The debate of which diaper cream is superior rages on in dermatology clinics, hospital wards, and daycares. The medical consensus is that a thick barrier is needed and should prevent irritants from coming into contact with the skin [24]. Most preferred diaper creams have zinc oxide in them at varying strengths. One pitfall is that some diaper creams can sometimes become gritty and cause physical irritation; thus having caregivers monitor for a gritty sensation during changes and switching to a different product can be helpful.

Concomitant infections with yeast are common; when this happens it usually involves the moist, dark, warm environment of the folds. Dermatologists generally prefer antifungal creams over powders as powders pose an inhalational risk to infants and can contribute to irritation with grittiness. Streptococcal and staphylococcal infections are both possible, and often require oral treatment [26]. Treatment for Gram negative and anaerobic bacteria in ulcerated skin can be approached with topical metronidazole, but care should be taken when making this diagnosis, as these organisms are common contaminants of the diaper area.

In the correct clinical context, the differential for diaper dermatitis may also include systemic conditions including zinc deficiency, (which can be seen in breast feeding patients with insufficient maternal zinc or premature infants on parenteral nutrition, and rarely as an inherited disorder), Langerhans cell histiocytosis (presents with seborrhea-like rash, in addition to erosive type rash in diaper area and flexures) and Coxsackie virus (or hand-foot-and-mouth; usually presents as a viral syndrome with fever and mouth sores) [26]. Other causes of diaper area rash are too extensive to address here, and can include early birthmarks, such as infantile hemangiomas, psoriasis, drug eruptions, staphylococcal scalded skin, or unusual ingestions. For example, a few case reports exist of erosive diaper dermatitis caused by children eating chocolate flavored laxatives intended for adults [27, 28].

In summary, diaper dermatitis is often multifactorial and a very common pediatric issue both in the inpatient and outpatient settings. Using all the necessary tools to provide protection, treat infections and allow the area to heal is key to successful treatment. It is important, when dealing with refractory diaper dermatitis, to keep less common diagnoses on the differential.

Answers

1. Langerhans cell histiocytosis, psoriasis, zinc deficiency.
2. Protecting from further irritation and repairing the barrier.

References

1. Lewis-Jones S. Quality of life and childhood atopic dermatitis: the misery of living with childhood eczema. Int J Clin Pract. 2006;60(8):984–92.
2. Wolter S, Price HN. Atopic dermatitis. Pediatr Clin North Am. 2014;61(2):241–60.
3. Eichenfield LF, Boguniewicz M, Simpson EL, Russell JJ, Block JK, Feldman SR, et al. Translating atopic dermatitis management guidelines into practice for primary care providers. Pediatrics. 2015;136(3):554–65.
4. Dabade TS, Davis DMR, Wetter DA, Hand JL, McEvoy MT, Pittelkow MR, et al. Wet dressing therapy in conjunction with topical corticosteroids is effective for rapid control of severe pediatric atopic dermatitis: experience with 218 patients over 30 years at Mayo Clinic. J Am Acad Dermatol. 2012;67(1):100–6.
5. Sidbury R, Davis DM, Cohen DE, Cordoro KM, Berger TG, Bergman JN, et al. Guidelines of care for the management of atopic dermatitis: section 3. Management and treatment with phototherapy and systemic agents. J Am Acad Dermatol. 2014;71(2):327–49.
6. Lang C, Cox M. Pediatric cutaneous bleach burns. Child Abuse Negl. 2013;37(7):485–8.
7. Sidbury R, Tom WL, Bergman JN, Cooper KD, Silverman RA, Berger TG, et al. Guidelines of care for the management of atopic dermatitis: section 4. Prevention of disease flares and use of adjunctive therapies and approaches. J Am Acad Dermatol. 2014;71(6):1218–33.
8. NIAID-Sponsored Expert Panel, Boyce JA, Assa'ad A, Burks AW, Jones SM, Sampson HA, et al. Guidelines for the diagnosis and management of food allergy in the United States: report of the NIAID-sponsored expert panel. J Allergy Clin Immunol. 2010;126(6):S1–58.
9. Paller AS, Mancini AJ. Hurwitz's clinical pediatric dermatology : a textbook of skin disorders of childhood and adolescence. 4th ed. Philadelphia: Elsevier/Saunders; 2011.
10. James WD, Berger TG, Elston DM. Andrews' diseases of the skin: clinical dermatology. 12th ed. Philadelphia: Elsevier; 2015. 968p.
11. Bhutani T, Hong J, Koo J. Contemporary diagnosis and management of psoriasis. 5th ed. Newtown: Handbooks in Healthcare; 2011.

12. Bolognia JL, Jorizzo JL, Schaffer JV. Dermatology. 3rd ed. Toronto: Elsevier; 2012. 2776p.
13. Jacob SE, Yang A, Herro E, Zhang C. Contact allergens in a pediatric population: association with atopic dermatitis and comparison with other north american referral centers. J Clin Aesthetic Dermatol. 2010;3(10):29–35.
14. Vongyer GA, Green C. Allergic contact dermatitis in children: has there been a change in allergens? Clin Exp Dermatol. 2015;40(1):31–4.
15. Zug KA, Pham AK, Belsito DV, DeKoven JG, DeLeo VA, Fowler JF, et al. Patch testing in children from 2005 to 2012: results from the North American contact dermatitis group. Dermat Contact Atopic Occup Drug. 2014;25(6):345–55.
16. Chang MW, Nakrani R. Six children with allergic contact dermatitis to methylisothiazolinone in wet wipes (baby wipes). Pediatrics. 2014;133(2):e434–8.
17. Climo MW, Yokoe DS, Warren DK, Perl TM, Bolon M, Herwaldt LA, et al. Effect of daily chlorhexidine bathing on hospital-acquired infection. N Engl J Med. 2013;368(6):533–42.
18. Milstone AM, Elward A, Song X, Zerr DM, Orscheln R, Speck K, et al. Daily chlorhexidine bathing to reduce bacteremia in critically ill children: a multicenter, cluster-randomized, two-period crossover trial. Lancet. 2013;381(9872):1099–106.
19. Noto MJ, Domenico HJ, Byrne DW, Talbot T, Rice TW, Bernard GR, et al. Chlorhexidine bathing and health care-associated infections: a randomized clinical trial. JAMA. 2015;313(4):369–78.
20. Cheng CE, Kroshinsky D. Iatrogenic skin injury in hospitalized patients. Clin Dermatol. 2011;29(6):622–32.
21. Eichenfield LF, Frieden IJ, Mathes EF, Zaenglein AL. Neonatal and infant dermatology. 3rd ed. Philadelphia: Saunders; 2014. 568p.
22. Williams KW, Milner JD, Freeman AF. Eosinophilia associated with disorders of immune deficiency or immune dysregulation. Immunol Allergy Clin North Am. 2015;35(3):523–44.
23. Goddard DS, Horn BN, McCalmont TH, Cordoro KM. Clinical update on graft-versus-host disease in children. Semin Cutan Med Surg. 2010;29(2):92–105.
24. Stamatas GN, Tierney NK. Diaper dermatitis: etiology, manifestations, prevention, and management. Pediatr Dermatol. 2014;31(1):1–7.
25. White CM, Gailey RA, Lippe S. Cholestyramine ointment to treat buttocks rash and anal excoriation in an infant. Ann Pharmacother. 1996;30(9):954–6.
26. Coughlin CC, Eichenfield LF, Frieden IJ. Diaper dermatitis: clinical characteristics and differential diagnosis. Pediatr Dermatol. 2014;31 Suppl 1:19–24.
27. Smith WA, Taintor AR, Kos L, Drolet B. Senna-containing laxative inducing blistering dermatitis in toddlers. Arch Dermatol. 2012;148(3):402–4.
28. Spiller HA, Winter ML, Weber JA, Krenzelok EP, Anderson DL, Ryan ML. Skin breakdown and blisters from senna-containing laxatives in young children. Ann Pharmacother. 2003;37(5):636–9.

Chapter 2
Viral Infections

Patrick McMahon and Robert James Smith

Abstract Cutaneous manifestations of viral infections in pediatric patients can provide the first critical clues to disease development. While often self-limiting, viral infections can cause serious morbidity and mortality in vulnerable pediatric populations. In this chapter, we review the clinical presentation, differential diagnosis and treatment of hand foot mouth disease, neonatal herpes simplex virus infection, disseminated varicella zoster in an immunocompromised patient and Lipschütz ulcers.

Keywords Viral exanthem • Coxsackievirus • Enterovirus • Herpes simplex virus • Varicella zoster virus • Epstein–Barr virus • Lipschütz ulcer • Acyclovir

Case 2.1

A 13-month-old female is admitted to the hospital for a severe flare of atopic dermatitis (AD). Her parents report that this flare began 2 days ago with a fever (T_{max} 101°F) and fussiness. She has been able to drink, but has been eating less solid foods. She has developed blisters and sores on the arms, legs, buttocks, and around her mouth. They especially noticed redness and sores within the areas affected by AD, including her antecubital and popliteal fossae. She has had both increased itching of the arms and legs as well as tenderness in some of the areas with open sores. Today, they noticed a few new bumps on the hands and feet. The patient has had mild AD since the age of 6 months that has been controlled well on low potency topical steroids until this flare. They have not applied medications or emollients since this flare began due to perceived discomfort upon attempted applications. The patient is otherwise healthy. There were no known sick contacts and no contact with active cold sores or herpes virus. However, today the mother began noticing painful

P. McMahon, MD (✉) • R.J. Smith, BS
Department of Pediatric Dermatology, The Children's Hospital of Philadelphia,
3550 Market Street, 2nd Floor, Philadelphia, PA 19104, USA

The Perelman School of Medicine at the University of Pennsylvania,
Philadelphia, PA 19104, USA
e-mail: mcmahonp@email.chop.edu

© Springer International Publishing Switzerland 2016
M. Hogeling (ed.), *Case-Based Inpatient Pediatric Dermatology*,
DOI 10.1007/978-3-319-31569-0_2

Fig. 2.1 Scattered vesicles
and erosions on legs with
accentuation in the
popliteal fossae

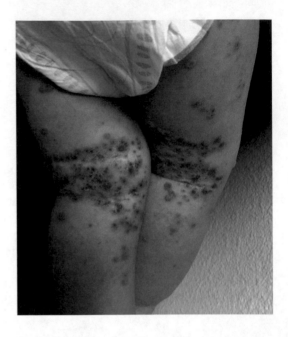

blisters on her own palms. On physical exam, the child appears nontoxic, but fussy
with scattered intact individual vesicles noted on the arms, legs, and buttocks; vesicles, crusting, and erosions around the mouth and within the antecubital and popliteal fossae; three vesicles noted on the soft palate and several papulovesicles on the
dorsal hands, dorsal feet and on the soles. The vesicles are mostly not clustered, but
in and around the scaly pink plaques of the antecubital and popliteal fossae the erosions appear accentuated and more concentrated (Fig. 2.1).

Questions

1. What is your differential diagnosis?
2. How would you treat the rash?
3. What are some delayed sequelae of this infection?

Presentation

Hand, foot, and mouth disease (HFMD) is a common pediatric illness due to enterovirus that typically presents with fever, painful erosions on the oral mucosa, and
small, gray-white, oval vesicles on the palms, soles, and buttocks [1]. While the
most common culprits of HFMD are Coxsackievirus A16 and enterovirus 71, starting in 2012, the Center for Disease Control reported a growing number of severe,
atypical cases of HFMD attributed to a different stain of the virus, Coxsackievirus
A6 (CVA6) [2]. In addition to classical HFMD symptoms of low-grade fever,

malaise, and gastrointestinal or respiratory complaints, patients with CVA6 often present with more extensive cutaneous lesions [1]. Outbreaks have been reported in Asia, Europe, and the United States [3, 4]. While classical HFMD affects children under the age of 6, CVA6 manifests in adults as well [4, 5]. Transmission occurs via oral or respiratory droplets with viral replications occurring in the pharynx and intestine. Subsequent viral amplification within the lymphatics results in viremia with distant multiorgan spread, including the skin.

The cutaneous manifestations of CVA6 infection are characterized by widespread vesiculobullous and erosive lesions extending beyond the palms and soles to include the trunk, extremities, and perioral region [1, 6]. A concurrent enanthem also consists of small vesicles and erosions on the oral mucosa. Perioral involvement may, in fact, be a hallmark of CVA6 infection [7]. In patients with a history of atopic dermatitis, as with the patient in presented case, lesions tend to concentrate in areas most affected by the individual's eczema, leading to the specific diagnosis of "eczema Coxsackium" or "eczema enteroviricum" [8, 9]. In these individuals, lesion morphology can appear quite similar to eczema herpeticum, except that in "eczema coxsackium" the vesicles tend to be less clustered and involvement of the palms and soles can be a clue that the patient has HFMD. Eruption patterns reveal a predilection for the virus to congregate in areas of previous trauma, friction or irritation, which may explain why disease severity is often worse on the palms, soles, and buttocks [1, 8].

Differential Diagnosis (Table 2.1)

The differential diagnosis for HFMD depends on the general presence or absence of cutaneous involvement. When there is only involvement of oral mucosa, the differential for these lesions includes orolabial HSV infection, aphthous stomatitis, and primary herpangina [8]. When there is widespread cutaneous involvement, other entities to consider within the differential for "eczema Coxsackium" include eczema herpeticum (HSV), varicella (VZV), disseminated zoster, bullous impetigo, erythema multiforme major, and bacterial superinfection of atopic dermatitis [5–8].

Diagnosis, Management, and Sequelae

Diagnosis of Coxsackie A6 HFMD is based primarily on clinical presentation. The diagnosis of an enteroviral infection can be confirmed via polymerase chain reaction (PCR) detection of the virus within the vesicle fluid, crusting or an erosion. For confirmation of the A6 serotype, nucleotide sequencing can be performed on PCR-positive specimens [1]. A skin biopsy is usually not necessary. If performed, it may reveal a spongiotic dermatitis, focal interface dermatitis with areas of subepidermal separation, and edema of the papillary dermis [1]. In patients with suspected "eczema Coxsackium," given the similarity in morphological appearance to eczema herpeticum, it is prudent to collect a sample of vesicular fluid for HSV PCR and consider empiric treatment with acyclovir if the eruption is severe [7].

Table 2.1 Differential diagnosis of viral exanthems by lesion morphology

Description of lesion morphology	Small, gray-white, oval vesicles on the palms, soles, and buttocks	Disseminated clustered, coalescing vesicles with surrounding erythema *in a neonate*	Dermatomal papulo-vesicular lesions	Disseminated papulo-vesicular lesions with crusting in various stages of development	Necrotic, painful, acute ulcer of the labia
Etiological category					
Infection/infestation	Eczema Coxsackium, eczema herpeticum, primary or disseminated VZV, bacterial superinfection of eczema	Neonatal HSV, disseminated VZV, Group B streptococcal infection, staphylococcal skin infection, toxoplasmosis, syphilis, rubella, cytomegalovirus	VZV, dermatomal HSV	Primary VZV, disseminated zoster, generalized HSV, enterovirus, scabies	HSV, syphilis, chancroid, HIV, tuberculosis, Lipschütz Ulcer (EBV, CMV)
Autoimmune	Linear IgA disease, bullous pemphigoid	Bullous mastocytosis		Guttate psoriasis, dermatitis herpetiformis	Behcet's disease, Crohn's disease, autoimmune bullous disease
Drug reaction					Fixed drug reaction
Other	Erythema multiforme (secondary to HSV or medication)		Contact dermatitis, burns, arthropod reaction	Kaposi's varicelliform eruption, papular urticaria, Langerhans cell histiocytosis, PLEVA	Trauma, contact dermatitis, pyoderma gangrenosum aphthous vulvar ulcer

The course of the illness is acute and self-limited. Treatment of concurrent atopic dermatitis with topical steroids and emollients may be indicated. Systemic symptoms typically resolve within a few days, and skin lesions resolve without scarring within days to weeks. Serious systemic complications in otherwise healthy patients are rare, but can include dehydration and viral meningoencephalitis. A known sequelae of CVA6 infection is delayed onychomadesis due to temporary arrest of the nail matrix, typically occurring 3–8 weeks after disease onset [6]. Patients typically experience full regrowth of their nails [9]. Patients may also experience desquamation of the palms and soles in the weeks following resolution of the vesicobullous eruption [1, 6].

Case 2.2

A 10-day-old male is admitted to the neonatal intensive care unit with fever, lethargy, and a widespread eruption. His parents report that he was born via normal spontaneous vaginal delivery at 39 weeks after an uncomplicated pregnancy. He was discharged home with his mother on day 2 of life and had been feeding well until yesterday when he began appearing excessively sleepy and refused to feed. Overnight, they noticed a small cluster of blisters on his abdomen. This morning he has several more blisters forming on his body, felt hot to the touch, and was found to have a temperature of 103°F. The mother has a remote history of genital herpes, but has not had any known active lesions for several years and, therefore, has not been on antiviral treatment recently. He was brought into the emergency department and underwent a full sepsis work-up for neonatal fever. Swabs were sent for viral and bacterial cultures from the vesicles on the skin. On physical exam, the child is found to be very irritable with widespread bright red clusters of erosions with scalloped borders on the abdomen, flanks, back, arms, legs, scalp, and buttocks. Upon close inspection he is also found to have intact clustered vesicles on the abdomen and an individual vesicopustule on the right forearm (Fig. 2.2).

Questions

1. What are the three types of presentation of this disease?
2. What is your differential diagnosis?
3. What is your treatment?

Presentation

Neonatal herpes simplex virus (HSV) is a herpetic infection that manifests within the first 28 days of life. While rare, with about 1500 cases annually, the infection carries significant morbidity and mortality [10]. Neonatal HSV can be transmitted

Fig. 2.2 Widespread
cropped erosions with
scalloped borders on the
torso of a neonate
(Photograph courtesy of
Paul Honig, M.D.)

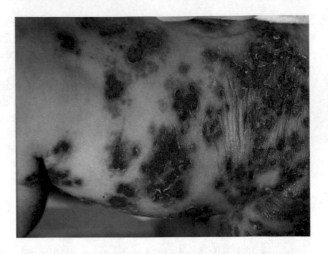

in three distinct periods: intrauterine, peripartum, and postnatal [11]. The majority
(85%) of neonatal HSV infection are acquired in the perinatal period when infants
are directly exposed to HSV infection in the mother's genital tract. An additional
10% of patients acquire the infection postnatally, typically via transmission from a
caretaker with HSV-1. The remaining 5% of patients acquire the infection through
intrauterine transmission [11].

For purposes of treatment and prognosis, neonatal HSV infections are divided
into three types: localized "skin, eye, and mouth" (SEM) disease, central nervous
system (CNS) disease, and disseminated disease. All three forms of neonatal HSV
can be caused by either HSV-1 or HSV-2, though HSV-2 infections have been associated with poorer outcomes [11].

Localized SEM disease accounts for 45% of neonatal HSV cases and classically
presents with clustered, coalescing small 2–4 mm vesicles on an erythematous base
[12]. Lesion morphology can also take the appearance of pustules, blisters, or ulcerations. While it can occur at any point within the first 6 weeks of life, lesions will typically manifest within the first 2 weeks [13]. Early signs of HSV infection of the eye
include excessive watering, conjunctival erythema, and crying from apparent eye pain.
Keratoconjunctivits from HSV can progress to chorioretinitis and cataracts, causing
permanent vision impairments [14]. HSV of the oropharyngeal cavity is characterized
by ulcerative lesions of the mouth, tongue, and palate. While benign appearing, treatment is critical to prevent progression to CNS or disseminated disease. If antiviral treatment is initiated prior to development of further disease, outcomes are favorable.

CNS neonatal herpes, also described as HSV meningoencephalitis, accounts for
1/3 of neonatal HSV infections [14]. It can occur through either hematogenous spread
from disseminated disease or localized retrograde spread from the nasopharynx and
olfactory nerves to the brain. CNS disease typically presents in the second or third
week of life and can occur with or without localized or disseminated diseases.
Clinical manifestations include seizures, irritability, poor feeding, tremors, full anterior fontanelles, and temperature instability [15]. Lumbar puncture for cerebrospinal

fluid [CSF] may appear normal early in the disease course, but classically shows a mononuclear cell pleocytosis, normal glucose, and mildly elevated protein. An electroencephalogram is often abnormal early in the disease course, showing multifocal periodic epileptiform discharges [11, 16]. Of note, without vesicular skin findings, it may be impossible to distinguish HSV meningoencephalitis from other forms of neonatal meningitis. If clinical and laboratory findings are suggestive or inconclusive for aseptic meningitis, treatment with acyclovir is recommended [17].

The least common form of neonatal HSV is disseminated disease, accounting for 25 % of cases. Disseminated illness can involve multiple organs, including the liver, lungs, and adrenals, in addition to CNS and/or SEM disease [14]. These neonates typically present in the first week of life with signs and symptoms of neonatal sepsis, including fever or hypothermia, irritability, poor feeding, lethargy, abdominal distension, and respiratory distress [11]. Disseminated disease progresses quickly, often resulting in respiratory failure, necrotizing enterocolitis, acute liver failure secondary to hepatitis, meningoencephalitis, and/or shock, similar to multiorgan involvement of bacterial sepsis. Since most (80 %) patients with disseminated illness have vesicular skin findings, the identification of skin findings can be significant for halting disease progress [14].

Differential Diagnosis

The differential diagnosis for vesicular skin findings in neonates includes other infectious etiologies, such as varicella zoster virus (VZV), enteroviral infection, group B streptococcal (GBS) infection, staphylococcal skin infection, listeriosis, and other congenital "TORCH" infection (toxoplasmosis, syphilis, rubella, cytomegalovirus) [12, 18]. The differential diagnosis also includes bullous mastocytosis, bullous impetigo, incontinentia pigmenti, and other blistering disorders.

Treatment and Management

Given the severity of disease progression, prompt recognition and treatment of neonatal herpes is of critical importance in infants with mucocutaneous vesicles, CNS abnormalities, or sepsis-like syndromes. Detection of HSV may be achieved through isolation of HSV in viral cell culture, detection of viral DNA via polymerase chain reaction (PCR), or rapid direct fluorescence antibody (DFA). However, negative cultures, PCR, or DFA cannot always rule out neonatal HSV. Alternatively, a Tzanck smear can be conducted to provide rapid diagnosis via visualization of multinucleated giant cells, though a positive result will not distinguish between HSV and VZV, and it may be unreliable due to interpreter variability [12].

Mortality exceeds 80 % in patients with untreated disseminated HSV disease, and serious morbidity can result, even with patients who receive early intervention [12]. The recommended antiviral treatment for suspected neonatal HSV is intravenous acyclovir [19]. Localized infections should be treated for a minimum of

14 days, while CNS and disseminated disease should be treated for a minimum of 21 days. Since the advent of antiviral therapy, mortality for CNS disease has declined from 85 to 29 % and for disseminated disease from 50 to 4 % [19–21]. Early treatment of localized disease effectively prevents the disease course from progressing to CNS or disseminated illness [22]. Following parenteral treatment, suppressive oral therapy of acyclovir should be administered for 6 months.

While approximately 20–30 % of pregnant women in the United States are infected with HSV-2, most neonates with HSV are born to mothers without a known prior history of the infection [12, 23]. Risk of maternal-fetal transmission is much higher [25–50 %] in women who acquire primary genital HSV during their pregnancy compared to women with long-standing HSV-2 infections who experience viral reactivation in their genital tract at term [<1 %] [24]. As such, infants born to mothers with high suspicion of primary HSV should be treated empirically [25].

Case 2.3

A 16-year-old female with a recent diagnosis of acute lymphoblastic leukemia (ALL) presents with spreading pink papulovesicles on the hands, arms, and now trunk. The lesions were first noticed 2 days ago on the bilateral forearms and have since spread. The patient is currently undergoing consolidation chemotherapy and is pancytopenic. She has been afebrile, denies pain or itching associated with these lesions, and denies having any lesions in the mouth or genital region. Besides the new diagnosis of ALL, the patient has no other past medical history and was fully immunized. Upon physical exam, she is tired, but well appearing and has scattered individual pink intact papules and papulovesicles accentuated on the bilateral arms and hands with limited involvement of the trunk and two papulovesicles noted on the buttocks. The lesions are in a linear distribution on the right forearm and some are crusted. Upon palpation of these lesions, the patient denies pain. There are not relevant findings in the oral or genital mucosae. Follow-up physical exam the following day revealed several new lesions on the trunk, arms, and legs, frank vesiculation of several lesions on the distal arms, and crusting of two lesions on the trunk. A diagnostic swab was sent from one of the vesicles (Fig. 2.3).

Questions

1. What are the differences in presentation of this virus for immunocompetent and immunosuppressed patients?
2. What is your differential diagnosis?
3. What is your treatment?

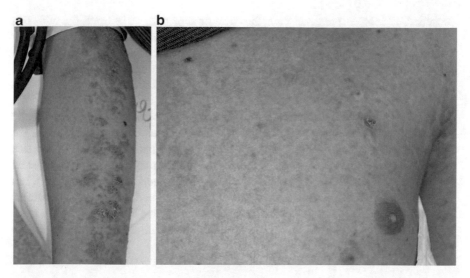

Fig. 2.3 Linear crusted papulovesicles on the arm (*left*), and scattered violaceous to pink papules on the chest (*right*)

Presentation

Varicella zoster virus (VZV) is a herpes virus that classically manifests as two different disease syndromes: primary infection (chickenpox) and reactivation ("herpes zoster" or "shingles") [26]. Primary infection is characterized by the presence of lesions in various stages of development on the face, trunk, and extremities that transition from macules to papules, pustules, vesicles, and crusts [26]. Lesions are typically most abundant on the central trunk and proximal upper extremities with relative sparing of the distal and lower extremities. Pruritus is an almost universal symptom associated with the lesions, along with fever and malaise [27]. Primary varicella is typically a self-limited disease in immunocompetent children, lasting about 7–10 days. However, complications can occur, such as bacterial superinfection, central nervous system (CNS) involvement (such as Reye's syndrome, Guillain–Barré, acute cerebral ataxia, and encephalitis), and varicella pneumonia [28, 29].

Primary VZV can have significant morbidity and mortality in immunocompromised hosts [30]. These patients may experience a prolonged febrile period, persistent viremia, and a more severe cutaneous presentation, often with purpuric or hemorrhagic lesions. These patients are also more likely to have involvement of the lungs, liver, and CNS [27]. Primary VZV can occur in previously immunized patients if their immunity has waned.

Herpes zoster is caused by reactivation of dormant varicella virus residing in the dorsal ganglia of previously infected patients. The zoster syndrome characterized by a painful, unilateral, dermatomal rash consisting of erythematous macules and papules, which then progress to vesicles, pustules, and crusts [31]. While the rash is preceded by intense pain and paresthesia in greater than 90 % of adults with this condition, lack of pain or limited pain is common in children with herpes zoster infections. Regional lymphadenopathy may or may not be present. Complications associated with zoster infections are rare in children, but include persistent regional pain, known as post-herpetic neuralgia [PHN], and ocular disease in patients with ophthalmic zoster [28].

As with primary VZV infection, the pain and rash associated with zoster may be more severe in immunocompromised patients [32]. Zoster can disseminate in up to 20–40 % of affected individuals [30]. Disseminated cutaneous zoster is defined as a patient having 20 or more vesicles *outside* of the primary affected and adjacent dermatomes. Visceral involvement of the lungs, liver, and CNS subsequently affect 10 % of these patients. Of note, as in the patient presented, atypical presentations and morphologies are possible in an immunocompromised host—specifically reactivated disseminated zoster is not always dermatomal in distribution, resembling acute varicella infection, and may be painless.

Differential Diagnosis

The differential for primary VZV infection includes other viral exanthems (generalized herpes simplex virus, disseminated herpes zoster, Kaposi's varicelliform eruption, or enterovirus), bacterial infections (bullous impetigo), drug eruptions (Stevens–Johnson syndrome), papular urticaria, pityriasis lichenoides et varioliformis acuta (PLEVA), Langerhans cell histiocytosis, guttate psoriasis, scabies, and dermatitis herpetiformis [26, 27]. In an immunocompromised host with atypical papular lesions, infectious etiologies such as disseminated candidiasis or atypical mycobacteria should also be considered.

The differential diagnosis for classical herpes zoster infections includes dermatomal HSV infections, contact dermatitis, localized viral or bacterial infections, arthropod reactions, and burns [26]. For disseminated zoster, the differential will be similar to that of disseminated primary varicella.

Diagnosis

Diagnosis is of primary varicella is often clinical based on characteristic lesion findings and a history of recent exposure to the virus within the previous 2–3 weeks. However, the diagnosis can also be confirmed through a number of laboratory methods [26]. The initial test of choice for patients with vesicular lesions in various stages of development is a viral PCR for HSV and VZV. Tzanck smear can also be done for rapid detection of multinuclear giant cells; however, the Tzanck will not distinguish VZV from herpes simplex virus [HSV] [12]. Viral culture and serological tests are alternative laboratory options. Serology may be helpful for distinguishing between primary VZV infection and reactivation, particularly when a history of primary chickenpox is uncertain [33].

Management

In healthy pediatric patients with uncomplicated primary varicella, treatment is symptomatic with antipyretics, antihistamines, and cool compresses [26]. In contrast, in immunocompromised pediatric patients, the treatment of choice for either primary varicella or herpes zoster is intravenous acyclovir [34, 35]. Early antiviral treatment prevents visceral dissemination of the virus [30, 32, 35]. To monitor the development of varicella complications in immunocompromised patients, laboratory evaluation should include a complete blood count, liver function tests, renal function test, and a chest radiograph [35]. Frequent clinical and laboratory evaluation should be rendered to monitor for the development of such complications. In otherwise immunocompetent patients who develop complications of varicella infections, such as pneumonia, encephalitis, or hepatitis, intravenous acyclovir is also indicated [35]. In rare cases of acyclovir-resistant VZV infections, foscarnet is the best drug available for treatment [36].

Prevention

Varicella is highly contagious, with infectivity rates in susceptible, unvaccinated patients ranging from 61 to 100 % [27]. The virus spreads in two forms: (1) via aerosolized droplets in the 2 days prior to appearance of skin lesions; and (2) via direct skin contact with the lesions 5–7 days after appearance of the rash. In immunocompromised hosts, the contagious period can last for several weeks. As such, patients in inpatient settings should be placed on droplet precautions. The live, attenuated varicella vaccine can safely be administered to children as young as 9 months and is highly effective, with prevention rates typically reaching 80–85 % [27].

Passive immunization with varicella zoster immunoglobin may be administrated to some susceptible groups who have been exposed to the virus. Eligible patients include immunocompromised children and adults for whom live vaccines are contraindicated, pregnant women, premature infants, and neonates whose mothers present with varicella infection in the period 5 days prior to 2 days after birth [37].

Case 2.4

A 15-year-old otherwise healthy female is admitted to the adolescent medicine service due to fever and severe, painful swelling and ulceration of the left labia majora and minora. The symptoms began 5 days ago with fever (T_{max} 102.5°F), mild swelling, and pain and have progressed to include ulceration and extreme dysuria prompting admission. The patient denies sexual activity. A preliminary work-up for sexually transmitted infections is negative including gonorrhea, chlamydia, human immunodeficiency virus (HIV), and a syphilis screen with rapid plasma reagin

(RPR). Bacterial swab from the left labial ulcer was negative as was HSV PCR. Monospot screening for Epstein–Barr virus (EBV) was positive and EBV serologies are pending. Upon physical exam, the well-appearing patient is noted to have left labial edema with mild pink erythema surrounding an ulceration between the labia major and minora with another more shallow ulceration noted on the inferior labia majora. Left inguinal lymphadenopathy is appreciated and painful to palpation. The physical exam overall is incredibly painful for the patient (Fig. 2.4).

Questions

1. What is your differential?
2. What is your management?

Presentation

Acute genital ulcers, also described as Lipschütz ulcers (LU), ulcus vulvae acutum, or nonsexual acute genital ulcers, are characterized by the sudden appearance of a single or multiple necrotic, painful ulcerations of the vulva, often in young prepubertal or adolescent women who are typically immunocompetent and nonsexually active [38, 39]. The ulceration is frequently large (>1 cm) and deep with a violaceous border, necrotic base, and grayish exudate or eschar. Ulcers can involve the labia minora, labia majora, perineum, and lower vagina. The ulceration are often preceded and accompanied by fever, dysuria, malaise, and inguinal lymphadenopathy [40, 41].

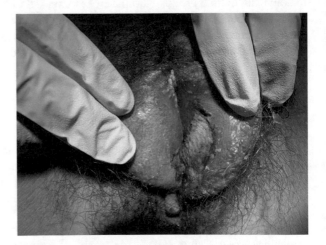

Fig. 2.4 Deep ulceration on the left labia with clean edges and minimal surrounding erythema (Photograph courtesy of Lara Wine-Lee, M.D., Ph.D.)

Differential Diagnosis

A Lipschütz ulcer is a diagnosis of exclusion. These lesions can be particularly distressing for patients, families, and providers, as their morphology and distribution can be mistaken for sexually transmitted infections and, consequently, as potential signs of abuse [39]. As such, their presence warrants a work-up to rule out multiple concerning etiologies. The diagnosis for LU should be distinguished from other venereal etiologies, such as herpes simplex virus (HSV), syphilis, and chancroid, as well as non-venereal infections, such as HIV, ulcerative tuberculosis, and paratyphoid fever. The differential also includes physical trauma, rheumatologic disease, such as Behcet's or Crohn's disease, pyoderma gangrenosum, fixed drug eruption, contact or irritant dermatitis, and autoimmune bullous diseases [39–41].

The cause of Lipschütz ulcers is most often linked to acute infection with EBV, though it has been associated with cytomegalovirus (CMV), influenza A virus, salmonella, toxoplasmosis, mycoplasma, Lyme, and paratyphoid fever virus [42]. In most patients, however, no specific etiology is ever identified [42, 43].

Diagnosis and Management

Initial work-up for these ulcers should first include a viral culture swab or polymerase chain reaction (PCR) for herpes simplex virus [HSV], as genital herpes simplex is the most common cause of genital ulcers. Serological tests for other causes of sexually transmitted genital ulcerations, such as syphilis, chancroid, chlamydia, and lymphogranuloma venereum, should also be performed, based on clinical suspicion and history. Serological testing for EBV is also indicated. Bacterial cultures of the ulcer should be obtained to assess for vulvar cellulitis and bacterial superinfection. Biopsy of the site is not initially indicated, as histology will appear nonspecific [40].

The lesion typically resolves without intervention within 2–6 weeks. Treatment entails reassurance, wound care in the form of Sitz baths, and pain control with acetaminophen, topical anesthetics, and systemic pain medications in severe cases or during painful physical exams [44]. Oral corticosteroids or high potency topical steroids may be used for the treatment of particularly painful, deep, or long-lasting ulcers [45]. Recurrence has been reported in up to a third of cases [40, 44].

References

1. Mathes EF, Oza V, Frieden IJ, Cordoro KM, Yagi S, Howard R, et al. "Eczema coxsackium" and unusual cutaneous findings in an enterovirus outbreak. Pediatrics [Internet]. 2013;132(1):e149–57.
2. McIntyre M, Stevens K, Todd R. Notes from the field. MMWR Morb Mortal Wkly Rep [serial online]. 2012;61(12):213–4.
3. Wu Y, Yeo A, Phoon MC, Tan EL, Poh CL, Quak SH, et al. The largest outbreak of hand; foot and mouth disease in Singapore in 2008: the role of enterovirus 71 and coxsackievirus A strains. Int J Infect Dis [Internet]. 2010 [cited 2015 Jul 6];14(12):e1076–81.

4. Ben-Chetrit E, Wiener-Well Y, Shulman LM, Cohen MJ, Elinav H, Sofer D, et al. Coxsackievirus A6-related hand foot and mouth disease: skin manifestations in a cluster of adult patients. J Clin Virol [Internet]. 2014;59(3):201–3.

5. Downing C, Ramirez-Fort MK, Doan HQ, Benoist F, Oberste MS, Khan F, et al. Coxsackievirus A6 associated hand, foot and mouth disease in adults: clinical presentation and review of the literature. J Clin Virol [Internet]. 2014 [cited 2015 Jun 7];60(4):381–6.

6. Wei S-H, Huang Y-P, Liu M-C, Tsou T-P, Lin H-C, Lin T-L, et al. An outbreak of coxsackievirus A6 hand, foot, and mouth disease associated with onychomadesis in Taiwan, 2010. BMC Infect Dis [Internet]. 2011 [cited 2015 Jul 6];11:346.

7. Flett K, Youngster I, Huang J, McAdam A, Sandora TJ, Rennick M, et al. Hand, foot, and mouth disease caused by coxsackievirus A6. Emerg Infect Dis. 2012;18(10):1702–4.

8. Lott JP, Liu K, Landry ML, Nix WA, Oberste MS, Bologna J, et al. Atypical hand-foot-and-mouth disease associated with coxsackievirus A6 infection. J Am Acad Dermatol [Internet]. 2013;69(5):736–41.

9. Feder HM, Bennett N, Modlin JF. Atypical hand, foot, and mouth disease: a vesiculobullous eruption caused by Coxsackie virus A6. Lancet Infect Dis [Internet]. 2014;14(1):83–6.

10. Flagg EW, Weinstock H. Incidence of neonatal herpes simplex virus infections in the United States, 2006. Pediatrics [Internet]. 2011 [cited 2015 Jul 14];127(1):e1–8.

11. Kimberlin DW. Neonatal herpes simplex infection. Clin Microbiol Rev [Internet]. 2004 [cited 2015 Jun 29];17(1):1–13.

12. Ladizinski B, Rukhman E, Lee KC. A 4-day-old neonate with a widespread vesicular rash. JAMA. 2013;310(9):9–10.

13. Kimberlin DW, editor. Herpes simplex. Red Book: 2015 Report of the Committee on Infectious Diseases. Elk Grove Village: American Academy of Pediatrics; 2015. p. 432.

14. Kimberlin DW. Herpes simplex virus infections of the newborn. Semin Perinatol [Internet]. 2007 [cited 2015 Jul 14];31(1):19–25.

15. Toth C, Harder S, Yager J. Neonatal herpes encephalitis: a case series and review of clinical presentation. Can J Neurol Sci [Internet]. 2003 [cited 2015 Jul 14];30(1):36–40.

16. Mizrahi EM, Tharp BR. A characteristic EEG pattern in neonatal herpes simplex encephalitis. Neurology [Internet]. 1982 [cited 2015 Jul 14];32(11):1215–20.

17. Long SS. In defense of empiric acyclovir therapy in certain neonates. J Pediatr [Internet]. 2008 [cited 2015 Jul 14];153(2):157–8.

18. Marquez L, Levy ML, Munoz FM, Palazzi DL. A report of three cases and review of intrauterine herpes simplex virus infection. Pediatr Infect Dis J [Internet]. 2011 [cited 2015 Jul 15];30(2):153–7.

19. Kimberlin DW, Lin CY, Jacobs RF, Powell DA, Corey L, Gruber WC, et al. Safety and efficacy of high-dose intravenous acyclovir in the management of neonatal herpes simplex virus infections. Pediatrics [Internet]. 2001 [cited 2015 Jun 29];108(2):230–8.

20. Whitley R, Arvin A, Prober C, Burchett S, Corey L, Powell D, et al. A controlled trial comparing vidarabine with acyclovir in neonatal herpes simplex virus infection. Infectious Diseases Collaborative Antiviral Study Group. N Engl J Med [Internet]. 1991 [cited 2015 Jul 14];324(7):444–9.

21. Pinninti SG, Kimberlin DW. Neonatal herpes simplex virus infections. Pediatr Clin North Am [Internet]. 2013 [cited 2015 Jun 5];60(2):351–65.

22. Turk DC, Swanson KS, Gatchel RJ. Predicting opioid misuse by chronic pain patients: a systematic review and literature synthesis. Clin J Pain [Internet]. 2008;24:497–508.

23. Caviness AC, Demmler GJ, Selwyn BJ. Clinical and laboratory features of neonatal herpes simplex virus infection: a case-control study. Pediatr Infect Dis J [Internet]. 2008 [cited 2015 Jul 14];27(5):425–30.

24. Corey L, Wald A. Maternal and Neonatal HSV Infections. N Engl J Med. 2009;361(14):1376–85.

25. ACOG Practice Bulletin. Clinical management guidelines for obstetrician-gynecologists. No. 82 June 2007. Management of herpes in pregnancy. Obstet Gynecol [Internet]. 2007 [cited 2015 Jul 15];109(6):1489–98.

26. McCrary ML, Severson J, Tyring SK. Varicella zoster virus. J Am Acad Dermatol [Internet]. 1999 [cited 2015 Jul 18];41(1):1–14; quiz 15–6.
27. Heininger U, Seward JF. Varicella. Lancet (London, England) [Internet]. 2006 [cited 2015 Jul 19];368(9544):1365–76.
28. Gilden DH, Kleinschmidt-DeMasters BK, LaGuardia JJ, Mahalingam R, Cohrs RJ. Neurologic complications of the reactivation of varicella-zoster virus. N Engl J Med [Internet]. 2000 [cited 2015 Jul 19];342(9):635–45.
29. Breuer J, Fifer H. Chickenpox. BMJ Clin Evid [Internet]. 2011 [cited 2015 Jul 19];2011.
30. Nyerges G, Meszner Z, Gyarmati E, Kerpel-Fronius S. Acyclovir prevents dissemination of varicella in immunocompromised children. J Infect Dis [Internet]. 1988 [cited 2015 Jul 18];157(2):309–13.
31. Wareham DW, Breuer J. Herpes zoster. BMJ [Internet]. 2007 [cited 2015 Jul 19];334(7605):1211–5.
32. Shepp DH, Dandliker PS, Meyers JD. Treatment of varicella-zoster virus infection in severely immunocompromised patients. A randomized comparison of acyclovir and vidarabine. N Engl J Med [Internet]. 1986 [cited 2015 Jul 19];314(4):208–12.
33. Petrun B, Williams V, Brice S. Disseminated varicella-zoster virus in an immunocompetent adult. Dermatol Online J [Internet]. 2015 [cited 2015 Jul 19];21(3).
34. Prober CG, Kirk LE, Keeney RE. Acyclovir therapy of chickenpox in immunosuppressed children—a collaborative study. J Pediatr [Internet]. 1982 [cited 2015 Jul 18];101(4):622–5.
35. Arvin AM. Antiviral therapy for varicella and herpes zoster. Semin Pediatr Infect Dis [Internet]. 2002 [cited 2015 Jul 18];13(1):12–21.
36. Piret J, Boivin G. Antiviral drug resistance in herpesviruses other than cytomegalovirus. Rev Med Virol [Internet]. 2014 [cited 2015 Jul 19];24(3):186–218.
37. Centers for Disease Control. A new product (VariZIG™) for postexposure prophylaxis of varicella available under an investigational new drug application expanded access protocol. MMWR Morb Mortal Wkly Rep [Internet]. 2006 [cited 2015 Jul 19];55:209–10.
38. Haidari G, MacMahon E, Tong CYW, White JA. Genital ulcers: it is not always simplex …. Int J STD AIDS [Internet]. 2015 [cited 2015 Jul 25];26(1):72–3.
39. Truchuelo MT, Vano-Galván S, Alcántara J, Pérez B, Jaén P. Lipschütz ulcers in twin sisters. Pediatr Dermatol [Internet]. 2012 [cited 2015 Jul 25];29(3):370–2.
40. Hernández-Núñez A, Córdoba S, Romero-Maté A, Miñano R, Sanz T, Borbujo J. Lipschütz [corrected] ulcers—four cases. Pediatr Dermatol [Internet]. 2008 [cited 2015 Jul 25];25(3):364–7.
41. Rosman IS, Berk DR, Bayliss SJ, White AJ, Merritt DF. Acute genital ulcers in nonsexually active young girls: case series, review of the literature, and evaluation and management recommendations. Pediatr Dermatol [Internet]. 2012 [cited 2015 Jul 25];29(2):147–53.
42. Farhi D, Wendling J, Molinari E, Raynal J, Carcelain G, Morand P, et al. Non-sexually related acute genital ulcers in 13 pubertal girls: a clinical and microbiological study. Arch Dermatol [Internet]. 2009 [cited 2015 Jul 25];145(1):38–45.
43. Deitch HR, Huppert J, Adams Hillard PJ. Unusual vulvar ulcerations in young adolescent females. J Pediatr Adolesc Gynecol [Internet]. 2004 [cited 2015 Jul 25];17(1):13–6.
44. Lehman JS, Bruce AJ, Wetter DA, Ferguson SB, Rogers RS. Reactive nonsexually related acute genital ulcers: review of cases evaluated at Mayo Clinic. J Am Acad Dermatol [Internet]. 2010 [cited 2015 Jul 25];63(1):44–51.
45. Dixit S, Bradford J, Fischer G. Management of nonsexually acquired genital ulceration using oral and topical corticosteroids followed by doxycycline prophylaxis. J Am Acad Dermatol [Internet]. 2013 [cited 2015 Jul 25];68(5):797–802.

Chapter 3
Bacterial Infections

Catalina Matiz and Emily Osier

Abstract Cutaneous manifestations of bacterial infections of pediatric patients can provide critical diagnostic information. Bacterial infections may cause significant morbidity and mortality in the pediatric population. Although often recognized by pediatricians, input from dermatologists may be helpful in assessing bullae, erosions, petechia, purpura, and morbilliform eruptions in systemically unwell children. In this chapter, we discuss the clinical presentation, differential diagnosis, and treatment of ecthyma gangrenosum, toxic shock syndrome, staphylococcal scalded skin syndrome, meningococcemia, and *methicillin-resistant Staphylococcus aureus* skin and soft tissue infections.

Keywords Community acquired *methicillin-resistant Staphylococcus aureus* • Skin infections in children • Ecthyma gangrenosum • *Pseudomona aeruginosa* • Toxic shock syndrome • *Neisseria meningitidis* • Meningococcemia

Case 3.1

History

A 2-year-old previously healthy female presented to the emergency department with a 3-week history of intermittent fevers, pallor, diffuse petechiae, and nose bleeds. Three days prior to presentation to the ED, she developed tender violaceous lesions on her arms, legs, and back (Figs. 3.1 and 3.2). The mother reported the lesions were initially red and had been turning more purple and tender over the last 2 days.

C. Matiz, MD (✉) • E. Osier
Division of Pediatric and Adolescent Dermatology, Department of Dermatology, University of California, San Diego, CA, USA

Division of Pediatric and Adolescent Dermatology, Department of Dermatology, Rady Children's Hospital, San Diego, CA, USA
e-mail: cmatiz@rchsd.org; ejosier@gmail.com

© Springer International Publishing Switzerland 2016   35
M. Hogeling (ed.), *Case-Based Inpatient Pediatric Dermatology*,
DOI 10.1007/978-3-319-31569-0_3

Physical Exam

Ill appearing child in mild distress. Her blood pressure is 101/56 mmHg, heart rate is 148/min, and her temperature is 40 °C. She has generalized pallor. No cervical lymphadenopathy. Conjunctiva is pale. Oral mucosa is dry and has few petechiae in her buccal mucosae and palate. She is tachycardic and has a systolic ejection murmur. Lungs are clear. Her liver is 2 cm below the costal margin and her spleen is not palpable.

On skin examination she had erythematous and violaceous nodules on back, extremities (Fig. 3.1), and buttocks as well as several necrotic plaques on arms and legs. She also has diffuse petechiae all over her body.

Laboratory Parameters

- White blood cell count 520 (4500–10,000 K/μL)
- Platelets 5000 (>150,000)
- LDH 2000 (110–295 U/L)
- Blood Culture-Positive for *Pseudomona aeruginosa*
- Tissue Culture-Positive for *Pseudomona aeruginosa*

Pathology

- Spongiosis
- Intraepidermal vesicle formation
- Diffuse dermal necrosis
- Subcuticular fat necrosis and extravasation of red blood cells
- Innumerable rod-shaped, filamentous bacteria, concentrated around blood vessels (Fig. 3.2)

Fig. 3.1 Erythematous indurated nodule with central necrotic plaque on left arm

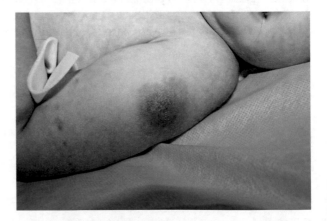

Fig. 3.2 Pathology.
Hematoxylin and Eosin.
×40. Innumerable
rod-shaped, filamentous
bacteria, concentrated
around blood vessels in
deep dermis

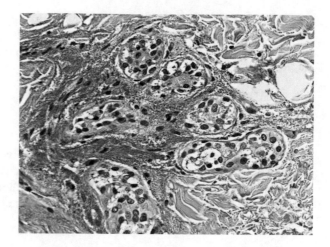

Questions

1. What is your differential diagnosis?
2. What treatments would you consider?

Answer

Ecthyma gangrenosum is a deep cutaneous infection with associated vasculitis affecting the media and adventitia of blood vessels which occurs from secondary seeding of a pathogen or direct inoculation through the skin. It is mainly caused by a systemic infection with *Pseudomona aeruginosa*, but other bacteria such as *E. Coli*, *Staphylococcus aureus*, *Streptococcus* species, candida species, herpes virus, and fungi (Mucor, Aspergillus, and fusarium species) have also been reported [1, 2]. It is classically described in patients with neutropenia either secondary to malignancy as in the case of this patient, or immunosuppressive therapy but cases in healthy individuals can also occur [3].

Clinically, the lesions start as red macules that evolve rapidly to papules or nodules and then become hemorrhagic and necrotic. Biopsy of the lesions typically shows a necrotizing vasculitis with scant neutrophilic infiltration and extensive bacillary infiltration of the perivascular region.

The differential diagnosis includes deep fungal infections, mycobacterial infection, paraneoplastic extensive necrotizing vasculitis, disseminated intravascular coagulation, calciphylaxis, septic emboli, loxoscelism, pyoderma gangrenosum, livedoid vasculopathy, antineutrophil cytoplasmic antibody (ANCA)-associated vasculitis, cutaneous necrotizing vasculitis as a manifestation of familial Mediterranean fever, and necrosis secondary to the use of vasoactive drugs [4].

The diagnosis is made on the basis of clinical history, characteristic lesions as well as tissue and blood cultures and findings on skin biopsy. If there is no known history of immunodeficiency or malignancy, a thorough immunodeficiency workup should be performed.

Treatment

These patients should be started on broad spectrum antibiotics such as fluoroquino-lones or B-lactam agents combined with an aminoglycoside. Use of aminoglyco-sides should be avoided in patients with renal insufficiency. Once culture and sensitivity results are back, antibiotics should be tailored to the specific pathogen causing the infection [5].

Case 3.2

History

A 9-year-old girl presented to the Emergency Department with fever and vomiting. The patient had a spider bite on the buttock for the last 3 days that had increased in size despite treatment with cephalexin. Her fever started the day prior to presentation and was up to 39 °C. This morning she continued to be febrile and started vomiting and has had one watery stool. The family also just noted a new rash on the trunk, arms, and legs.

Physical Exam

On exam, the patient is lethargic and febrile, and ill appearing. Her blood pressure is 60/40 mmHg, temperature is 39 °C, and heart rate is 150/min.

Head and neck exam is notable for conjunctival injection that includes the limbus, no discharge noted. Lips are dry without cracking; the tongue is smooth and red. Shotty anterior cervical adenopathy is appreciated. The patient is tachycardic with a systolic flow murmur, 2+ pulses, and clear lung fields. The liver is palpable below the costal margin, no splenomegaly, normal bowel sounds. There is a 3 cm indurated furuncle noted on the right buttock with central pustule. The patient has an erythematous macu-lopapular eruption on the trunk and extremities sparing the palms and soles (Fig. 3.3).

Laboratory Parameters

- White blood cell count 14,000/μL
- 72 % segmented neutrophils
- 20 % lymphocytes

Fig. 3.3 Erythematous macules and edematous papules and plaques on abdomen and thighs

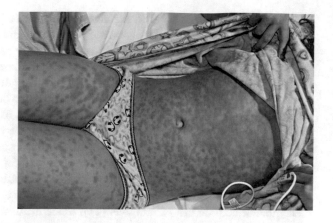

- Hemoglobin 12 g/dL
- Platelets 530,000/μL
- Creatinine 1.2 mg/dL
- ALT 85 units/dL
- AST 70 units/dL
- Blood and skin cultures pending

Questions

1. What is the differential diagnosis?
2. What are the most likely causative organisms?
3. What is the appropriate treatment?
4. What is the expected course?

Answers

Toxic shock syndrome (TSS) is a serious and under-recognized [6] systemic reaction to infection with either *Staphylococcus aureus* or *Streptococcus pyogenes*. While a bacterial infection is the inciting factor, it is not sepsis that causes the systemic symptoms but rather the bacterial production of superantigens [7]. *S. aureus* has the ability to produce enterotoxins responsible for toxic shock syndrome, including toxic shock syndrome toxin-1 (TSST-1), and enterotoxins-a, b, or c [7, 8], and *S. pyogenes* produces M proteins capable of acting as superantigens [7]. Both staphylococcal and streptococcal superantigens are able to cross-link the T-cell receptor with the MHC-II complex which leads to excessive T cell activation, activating 20–30 % of T cells versus the usual 0.001 % of T cells that are activated in a normal immune response [9]. This activation in turn leads to overwhelming cytokine production and the resultant systemic symptoms [7, 9].

The diagnostic criteria for TSS includes the presence of fever, rash, hypotension, and involvement of three or more organ systems, including gastrointestinal, mucosal, renal, hepatic, hematologic, or nervous systems. The patient described is febrile, hypotensive, has an ill-defined rash, and has compromise of her liver and kidney function which fulfills the criteria for TSS [10, 11]. Desquamation of the palms and soles following the acute phase is an additional criterion but is not normally identified when the diagnosis is made. A definite case of TSS has all criteria, and a probable case lacks only one criterion [10, 11]. TSS caused by *S. aureus* has somewhat different diagnostic criteria compared with streptococcal toxic shock syndrome (STSS). A diagnosis of STSS is made in the presence of *S. pyogenes* obtained from a normally sterile site in addition to the presence of fever, hypotension, and rash [9].

In the 1980s, there was an epidemic of TSS in young women associated with menstruation and the use of tampons [11]. Since then, with changes to menstrual care products, the rate of TSS has stabilized and there are now as many menstrual as non-menstrual cases. The current incidence of streptococcal TSS is equal to that of staphylococcal TSS [12, 13].

Differential Diagnosis

The differential diagnosis of toxic shock syndrome includes bacterial sepsis, systemic immune response syndrome, and Kawasaki disease with shock syndrome. There is considerable overlap in the symptoms of toxic shock syndrome and Kawasaki disease with shock syndrome, a variant of Kawasaki Disease (KD), including the presence of fever, conjunctivitis, mucous membrane erythema, rash, and hypotension [14]. In a comparative retrospective cohort review, patients with TSS were more likely to have elevated creatinine levels while patients with KD were more likely to have cardiac abnormalities on echocardiography [14].

Treatment

Treatment of TSS includes antibiotic treatment of the causative organism, immuno-modulating therapy and supportive care with IV fluids and vasopressors [7, 15]. Patients with TSS may be presumed to have an infection or be colonized with *S. aureus,* yet blood cultures are frequently negative [9]. Antibiotic choice empirically should include a penicillin and coverage for methicillin-resistant staphylococcus aureus until culture results are available. Methicillin-resistant *S. aureus* (MRSA) is a possible cause although less commonly reported than superantigen producing strains of methicillin-sensitive *S. aureus* [7]. The younger age range of patients who contract TSS, median age 21.4 years old [16], is postulated to be due to the lack of antibodies produced against superantigens by younger patients [7, 9]. Treatment with IVIg can provide antibodies to the causative superantigens and improve survival [7, 9, 12, 15]. There is speculation that the use of clindamycin, in addition to a penicillin for patients with STSS, further attenuates the cytokine storm by decreasing bacterial protein production as it blocks the 50S ribosome of Gram-positive bacteria [7, 12].

The course of TSS can have devastating results, with a mortality rate ranging from 3.2% [17] to 16% [12]. The morbidities of TSS can include ischemia of the extremities and organ failure, specifically renal, myocardial, or pulmonary dysfunction. Desquamation of the palms and soles is expected 1–3 weeks after symptom onset [7, 11]. Patients with staphylococcal TSS can be triggered by their nasopharyngeal or vaginal colonization of superantigen producing TSS. Attempts at decolonization of the family should be considered as patients have been reported with recurrent TSS despite a lack of active infection [18].

Case 3.3

History

A 3-week-old full-term male neonate was transferred from routine newborn care to the neonatal intensive care unit for evaluation and treatment of a new rash. The patient was the product of an uncomplicated pregnancy and delivery and was previously healthy, without a history of eczema. He developed an erythematous eruption on the neck 5 days prior to presentation. The eruption spread to the face and upper trunk. The parents applied topical emollients without improvement. The pediatrician evaluated the infant, noting a fever to 38.2 °C and drainage from an erythematous umbilical area. The family reported his 3-year-old brother had a skin infection with blisters and fluid drainage on the arm.

Physical Exam

On exam, the patient was well appearing with diffuse erythroderma. The periumbilical area had moderate erythema. There was maceration and superficial desquamation of the right scalp, neck, axillae, inguinal folds, perianal area, and inferior scrotum as well as several flaccid intact bullae on the upper and lower extremities (Fig. 3.4).

Laboratory Parameters

- White blood cell count: 6600/µL
- Hemoglobin 11.8 g/dL
- Normal comprehensive metabolic panel
- Normal urinalysis

Fig. 3.4 Neonate with diffuse erythroderma, *yellow* crusting and erythema of periorbital and perioral skin. Superficial desquamation noted on chest and neck

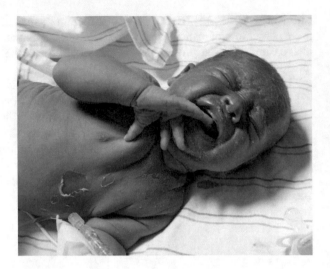

- Viral culture: negative
- Tzanck smear: negative
- Wound cultures from the neck, perianal, and umbilical skin: *Staphylococcus aureus*, methicillin sensitive

Questions

1. What is the differential diagnosis?
2. What is the preferred treatment for this condition?

Answers

Staphylococcal scalded skin syndrome (SSSS) is a blistering skin condition most frequently seen in children under 5 years of age, caused by *Staphylococcus aureus* subtypes that produce an exfoliating toxin. Patients typically present with an initial area of erythema around the eyes, mouth, or umbilicus. They progress to more generalized erythema and bullae formation [19].

Both methicillin-sensitive and methicillin-resistant strains of *S. aureus* have been implicated in SSSS [20]. *S. aureus* phage group II, types 71 and 55, produce the exotoxins exfoliative toxin A or exfoliative toxin B. These exotoxins target desmoglein-1 in the stratum granulosum of the superficial epidermis, which leads to bullae formation and desquamation [20]. Because of the fragility of the epidermis, patients have a positive Nikolsky's sign (lesional extension and shearing of skin that results from lateral pressure applied to the normal-appearing skin at the periphery of a lesion) on physical examination [19, 20].

Neonates and patients with impaired kidney function are at a higher risk for more severe disease and poorer outcome, as they are thought to be unable to efficiently clear the toxin [20]. A skin biopsy will show sub-corneal intraepidermal cleavage without inflammation or necrotic keratinocytes, but this is usually not needed [20, 21].

Differential Diagnosis

The differential diagnosis of a neonate with a blistering skin eruption includes toxic epidermal necrolysis (TEN), human enterovirus infection (specifically coxsackie virus and enterovirus 71), and less likely drug reaction with eosinophilia and systemic symptoms syndrome (DRESS), and staphylococcal toxic shock syndrome [8]. TEN is differentiated by the presence of mucosal involvement and, on biopsy, subepidermal cleavage [21]. DRESS is a drug-mediated hypersensitivity reaction most commonly associated with antiepileptic drugs that begins with fever prior to an erythematous eruption that can blister [22]. Staphylococcal toxic shock syndrome is also caused by an exfoliating exotoxin but has systemic instability as well as petechiae or desquamation of the palms and soles [8].

Treatment

Once the diagnosis is made the patient should be started on IV penicillinase-resistant penicillin and clindamycin as empiric treatment until culture susceptibility data are available to guide proper antibiotic therapy [23]. Supportive care is essential including monitoring of fluid and electrolyte status [19]. Outbreaks of SSSS have been reported in neonatal units [24], in which case identification of the causal carrier is important to prevent additional cases. Because of the superficial location of the blister within the epidermis, healing without scar is expected [20, 21]. Application of bland emollients such as petrolatum is recommended for the skin care of this patients.

In this case, the older brother also had a skin infection that was consistent with bullous impetigo. Decolonization of the family with intranasal mupirocin and dilute bleach baths was recommended [25].

Case 3.4

History

A 17-month-old boy was admitted to the children's hospital for fever, vomiting, and a rash. For 2 days prior to admission, he had rhinorrhea but was otherwise well. The evening prior to admission, he had a fever of 103.5 F and later started vomiting.

Overnight, he developed a rash on the legs and stomach that progressed to the arms. He was taken to the emergency department and subsequently admitted to the hospital. He received ceftriaxone and intravenous fluids after blood cultures were drawn.

Physical Exam

The patient was febrile and irritable but awake. He initially had a morbilliform eruption on the arms and trunk in the emergency department that resolved within approximately 24 h. After admission, there were scattered erythematous crusted papules and hemorrhagic purpuric macules on the arms, legs, and buttocks—including the palms and soles (Fig. 3.5). A stellate purpuric macule was noted on the buttocks (Fig. 3.6). There were scattered petechiae on the legs.

Laboratory Results

- White blood cell count: 26,400/µL
- Segmented neutrophils 53 %
- Banded neutrophils 23 %
- Platelets 226,000/µL
- aPTT 37 s
- PT 16.8 s
- INR 1.4
- Fibrinogen: 745 mg/dL
- D-Dimer 981

Fig. 3.5 Pink papules and violaceous angulated macules and papules and scattered petechiae on legs and buttocks

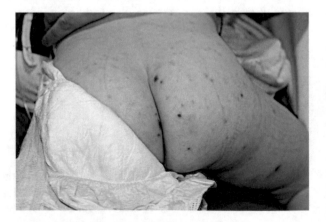

Fig. 3.6 Angulated deep *red* macule on dorsum of foot

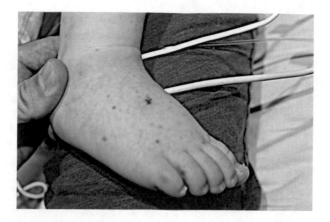

Questions

1. What is the differential diagnosis?
2. What is purpura fulminans?
3. What is the role for post-exposure prophylaxis?

Answers

The most commonly reported conditions caused by the Gram-negative bacteria *Neisseria meningitidis* are meningococcemia and meningococcal meningitis [26]. This patient was diagnosed with meningococcemia after the blood culture returned positive for *N. meningitidis*, serogroup B. The varying polysaccharide structures of *N. meningitidis* capsules identify the bacterial serogroup. Capsular serogroups A, C, W-135, and Y are responsible for causing the majority of meningococcal disease and are targeted by routinely administered vaccines [26, 27]. Following recent outbreaks on college campuses, a vaccine against serogroup B is available for those at increased risk [27]. *N. meningitidis* colonizes the human upper respiratory tract in about one-tenth of people and transmission occurs by saliva or respiratory droplets [26]. Invasive disease results if the bacteria penetrate into the bloodstream and/or meninges. In patients with invasive meningococcal disease, mortality rates have been reported from 10 to 40 % [26, 28]. The morbidities of meningococcal infection can include brain damage, deafness, renal failure, and extremity amputation [28].

Other than meningococcemia, the differential diagnosis of a purpuric eruption in a febrile child includes *Streptococcus pyogenes* infection, Rocky Mountain spotted fever, epidemic typhus, Henoch–Schönlein purpura, acute hemorrhage edema, vasculitic drug reaction, rat bite fever, atypical measles, parvovirus B19, and numerous bacterial, viral, or fungal causes of septicemia [29]. The morphology of the stellate purpuric lesion on the buttock was consistent with previously reported cases of *N.*

meningitidis infections [29]. The correct diagnosis was supported by the acute and simultaneous appearance of fever and petechial and purpuric eruption and was confirmed by a positive blood culture.

Purpura fulminans, which was not present in this case, is a rapidly progressive purpura due to hemorrhagic necrosis of the skin [30]. It occurs most often in acute bacteremia with *N. meningitidis, S. pyogenes, S. pneumoniae, and S. aureus,* and in patients with hereditary defects in protein C and S. The pathogenesis of purpura fulminans relates to systemic inflammation, endothelial dysfunction, activation of the clotting and complements cascades all leading to disseminated intravascular coagulation. Cases can have thrombosis in tissues other than the skin leading to muscle necrosis and multi-organ failure [30].

Treatment and Prophylaxis

When a patient presents with fever, purpuric and petechial lesions, meningococcemia should be highly considered. A blood culture should be performed and the patient should be started immediately on systemic antibiotics such as third-generation cephalosporins. Waiting to perform a lumbar puncture should not delay antibiotic administration.

It is common for patients with meningococcal disease to present in shock and for this reason they should be managed in a tertiary care medical facility. Adequate management with vasopressors and fluids is required in most cases.

Once the patient has been identified as having meningococcal disease, the public health authorities should be notified and attention should be paid to post-exposure prophylactic treatment of exposed individuals [31]. There have been cases of meningococcemia in health care workers who did not receive appropriate prophylaxis [31]. Treatment with either rifampin, ceftriaxone, ciprofloxacin, or azithromycin should be initiated within 24 h of the patient being diagnosed with meningococcal disease [31, 32]. Close contacts, such as household members, child-care workers and attendees, and health care workers exposed to a patient's oral secretions should be treated [31, 32].

Case 3.5

History

A 16-month-old female is brought to the emergency department by her mother for a 9-day history of two "spider bites" on her thigh that were getting larger, tender, and hotter despite being treated with cephalexin for the past 4 days by her pediatrician. She also started developing fever in the last 2 days. The mother reported there have been other family members with similar lesions at different points in time. The mother works in a small hospital as a medical assistant. There are no pets at home.

Physical Exam

The patient is febrile at 103.5 F. She is awake and alert.

Her heart rate is 120/min. Her blood pressure is 102/65.

On skin exam she has two indurated, erythematous, edematous, and hot round plaques on her right leg (Fig. 3.7). She has enlarged lymph nodes on her right inguinal region.

Laboratory Results

- White blood cell count 15,000/μL
- Segmented neutrophils 80 %
- Wound Culture: Methicillin-resistant *Staphylococcus aureus*
- Blood culture: Methicillin-resistant *Staphylococcus aureus*

Questions

1. What is the diagnosis?
2. What are the risk factors for this patient?
3. What is the recommended treatment?

Fig. 3.7 Erythematous, edematous, and crusted plaques on right leg

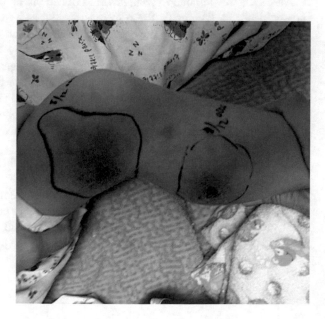

Answers

Staphyloccocus aureus is the most common cultured pathogen causing superficial skin and soft tissue infections (infections that are localized to epidermis, dermis, or both). In children, this bacteria accounts for ¼ of the outpatient office visits and emergency department encounters [33].

With the emergence of Methicillin-resistant *Staphylococcus aureus* (MRSA) in the United States the number of cases has dramatically increased specially for skin abscesses. The gene responsible for antibacterial resistance is the MecA gene encoded by the mobile genetic element, staphylococcal cassette chromosome (SSC) which encodes an altered penicillin binding protein [34]. Other important virulent factors of CA-MRSA include the presence of leukocidins such us Panto Vanlentine Leukocidin (PV), which has been associated with deep tissue infections as well as necrotizing pneumonia [35]. Other important virulent factors include α type phenol-soluble modulins (PSM) and type I argine catabolic mobile element (ACME) which promotes growth and survival of clone US300 within the skin and enables this bacteria to colonize human skin [36].

Cellulitis is an acute superficial skin infection that affects the dermis and subcutaneous tissue. Clinically, the skin is erythematous, edematous, and tender and has spreading irregular borders (Fig. 3.7). The most common pathogen causing this type of infection has been *Streptococcus pyogenes,* but with the emergence of CA-MRSA, this bacterial has become a common cause of cellulitis specially if associated to furuncles and abscesses. In certain occasions, the clinical impression of cellulitis could be difficult to differentiate from an abscess and this distinction is of importance as it can change the clinical management [37].

Abscesses are inflamed, "walled-off" collections of purulent exudate that are mostly localized. Clinically, these lesions present as a fluctuant, tender, firm erythematous nodules that may have purulent discharge and occasionally can be confused for a "spider bite." They are mainly caused by CA-MRSA followed by CA-MSSA and less likely *Proteus Mirabilis* and *S. pyogenes* [38].

Skin cultures in patients with suspected cellulitis are rarely positive and blood cultures in uncomplicated cases are positive less than 1 % of the time [39]. If the patient is sick and has systemic symptoms, the likelihood for a positive culture is about 12.5 % [39]. When the lesion is purulent as in an abscess, culture of the lesion is recommended to guide antibiotic therapy.

Some authors postulate the use of ultrasound to differentiate cases of cellulitis form an abscess if the diagnosis in question [37].

Populations at risk for CA-MRSA infections include neonates in intensive care units, athletes in contact sports, patients with a family or personal history of MRSA SSTI, patients in contact with health care facilities and personnel, patients with HIV, and patients in urban underserved communities [38].

Treatment

Recent recommendations suggest treating uncomplicated non-purulent superficial skin and soft tissue (SSTI) with a B-lactam antibiotic that covers for streptococci and MSSA [25]. If there is a failure to the initial empiric therapy as it occurred in this patient, coverage for CAMRSA should be undertaken. If the patient is toxic, which rarely occurs in patients with cellulitis unless they have a weakened immune system, they should be admitted to the hospital and treated with IV antibiotics such us clindamycin, vancomycin, linezolid, daptomycin, or telavancin.

If the lesion is purulent (abscess), the recommended therapy is incision and drainage alone in healthy children. If the patient has a history of immunodeficiency, the presence of any systemic symptoms of infection or failure to respond to I&D alone, systemic antibiotic therapy against MRSA is recommended [25].

References

1. Long SS, Pickering LK, Charles G. Principles and practice of pediatric infectious diseases. 4th ed. Philadelphia: Elsevier; 2012. p. 550.
2. Pathak A, Singh P, Yadav Y, Dhaneria M. Ecthyma gangrenosum in a neonate: not always pseudomonas. BMJ Case Rep. 2013; doi:10.1136/bcr-2013-009287
3. Cohen N, Capua T, Bilavsky E, Dias-Polak H, Levin D, Grisaru-Soen G. Ecthyma gangrenosum skin lesions in previously healthy children. Acta Paediatr. 2015;104(3):e134–8.
4. Vaiman M, Lazarovitch T, Heller L, Lotan G. Ecthyma gangrenosum and ecthyma-like lesions: review article. Eur J Clin Microbiol Infect Dis. 2015;34(4):633–9.
5. Long SS, Pickering LK, Charles G. Principles and practice of pediatric infectious diseases. 4th ed. Philadelphia: Elsevier; 2012. p. 845.
6. Curtis N. Toxic shock syndrome: under-recognised and under-treated? Arch Dis Child. 2014;99(12):1062–4.
7. Low DE. Toxic shock syndrome: major advances in pathogenesis, but not treatment. Crit Care Clin. 2013;29(3):651–75.
8. Chi C-Y, Wang S-M, Lin H C, Liu C-C. A clinical and microbiological comparison of Staphylococcus aureus toxic shock and scalded skin syndromes in children. Clin Infect Dis. 2006;42(2):181–5.
9. Kulhankova K, King J, Salgado-Pabon W. Staphylococcal toxic shock syndrome: superantigen-mediated enhancement of endotoxin shock and adaptive immune suppression. Immunol Res. 2014;59(1–3):182–7.
10. Wharton M, Chorba TL, Vogt RL, Morse DL, Buehler JW. Case definitions for public health surveillance. MMWR Recomm Rep. 1990;39:1–43.
11. Reingold AL, Hargrett NT, Shands KN, Dan BB, Schmid GP, Stickland BY. Toxic shock syndrome surveillance in the United States, 1980–1981. Ann Intern Med. 1982;96:875–80.
12. Adalat S, Dawson T, Hackett SJ, Clark JE. Toxic shock syndrome surveillance in UK children. Arch Dis Child. 2014;99(12):1078–82.
13. Smit MA, Nyquist AC, Todd JK. Infectious shock and toxic shock syndrome diagnoses in hospitals, Colorado, USA. Emerg Infect Dis. 2013;19(11):1855–8.
14. Lin YJ, Cheng MC, Lo MH, Chien SJ. Early differentiation of Kawasaki disease shock syndrome and toxic shock syndrome in a pediatric intensive care unit. Pediatr Infect Dis J. 2015;34(11):1163–7.

15. Linner A, Darenberg J, Sjolin J, Henriques-Normark B, Norrby-Teglund A. Clinical efficacy of polyspecific intravenous immunoglobulin therapy in patients with streptococcal toxic shock syndrome: a comparative observational study. Clin Infect Dis. 2014;59(6):851–7.

16. DeVries AS, Lesher L, Schlievert PM, Rogers T, Villaume LG, Danila R, et al. Staphylococcal toxic shock syndrome 2000–2006: epidemiology, clinical features, and molecular characteristics. PLoS One. 2011;6(8), e22997.

17. Centers for Disease Control and Prevention. Nosocomial group A streptococcal infections associated with asymptomatic health-care workers—Maryland and California, 1997. Morb Mortal Wkly Rep. 1999;48(8):163–6.

18. Tremlett W, Michie C, Kenol B, van der Bijl S. Recurrent menstrual toxic shock syndrome with and without tampons in an adolescent. Pediatr Infect Dis J. 2014;33(7):783–5.

19. Oranje AP, de Waard-van der Spek FB. Recent developments in the management of common childhood skin infections. J Infect. 2015;71 Suppl 1:S76–9.

20. Handler MZ, Schwartz RA. Staphylococcal scalded skin syndrome: diagnosis and management in children and adults. J Eur Acad Dermatol Venereol. 2014;28(11):1418–23.

21. Amagai M, Matsuyoshi N, Wang ZH, Andl C, Stanley JR. Toxin in bullous impetigo and staphylococcal scalded-skin syndrome targets desmoglein 1. Nat Med. 2000;6(11):1275–7.

22. Avancini J, Maragno L, Santi CG, Criado PR. Drug reaction with eosinophilia and systemic symptoms/drug-induced hypersensitivity syndrome: clinical features of 27 patients. Clin Exp Dermatol. 2015;40(8):851–9.

23. Braunstein I, Wanat KA, Abuabara K, McGowan KL, Yan AC, Treat JR. Antibiotic sensitivity and resistance patterns in pediatric staphylococcal scalded skin syndrome. Pediatr Dermatol. 2014;31(3):305–8.

24. Paranthaman K, Bentley A, Milne LM, Kearns A, Loader S, Thomas A, et al. Nosocomial outbreak of staphyloccocal scalded skin syndrome in neonates in England, December 2012 to March 2013. Euro Surveill. 2014;19(33):pii: 20880.

25. Stevens DL, Bisno AL, Chambers HF, Dellinger EP, Goldstein EJ, Gorbach SL. Practice guidelines for the diagnosis and management of skin and soft tissue infections: 2014 update by the Infectious Diseases Society of America. Clin Infect Dis. 2014;59(2):e10–52.

26. Gianchecchi E, Torelli A, Piccini G, Piccirella S, Montomoli E. Neisseria meningitidis infection: who, when and where? Expert Rev Anti Infect Ther. 2015;24:1–15.

27. Folaranmi T, Rubin L, Martin SW, Patel M, MacNeil JR. Use of serogroup B meningococcal vaccines in persons aged ≥10 years at increased risk for serogroup B meningococcal disease: recommendations of the advisory committee on immunization practices, 2015. MMWR Morb Mortal Wkly Rep. 2015;64(22):608–12.

28. Rosenstein NE, Perkins BA, Stephens DA, Popovic T, Hughes JM. Meningococcal disease. N Engl J Med. 2001;344(18):1378–88.

29. Baselga E, Drolet BA, Esterly NB. Purpura in infants and children. J Am Acad Dermatol. 1997;37(5 Pt 1):673–705.

30. Chalmers E, Cooper P, Forman K, Grimley C, Khair K, Minford A, et al. Purpura fulminans: recognition, diagnosis and management. Arch Dis Child. 2011;96:1066–71.

31. Materna B, Harriman K, Rosenberg J, Shusterman D, Windham G, Atwell J, et al. Occupational Transmission of Neisseria meningitides, California, 2009. MMWR Morb Mortal Wkly Rep. 2010;59(45):1480–3.

32. Siegel JD, Rhinehart E, Jackson M, Chiarello L. Health Care Infection Control Practices Advisory Committee. 2007 guideline for isolation precautions: preventing transmission of infectious agents in health care settings. Am J Infect Control. 2007;35(10 suppl 2):S65–164.

33. Moet GJ, Jones RN, Biedenbach DJ, et al. Contemporary causes of skin and soft tissue infections in North America, Latin America, and Europe: report from the SENTRY Antimicrobial Surveillance Program (1998–2004). Diagn Microbiol Infect Dis. 2007;57(1):7–13.

34. Britton PN, Andresen DN. Paediatric community-associated Staphylococcus aureus: a retrospective cohort study. J Paediatr Child Health. 2013;49(9):754–9.

35. Shallcross LJ, Fragaszy E, Johnson AM, et al. The role of the Panton-Valentine leucocidin toxin in staphylococcal disease: a systematic review and meta-analysis. Lancet Infect Dis. 2012;13(1):43–54.
36. Jahamy H, Ganga R, Al Raiy B, et al. *Staphylococcus aureus* skin/soft-tissue infections: the impact of SCCmec type and Panton-Valentine leukocidin. Scand J Infect Dis. 2008;40:601–6.
37. Fenster DB, Renny MH, Ng C, Roskind CG. Scratching the surface: a review of skin and soft tissue infections in children. Curr Opin Pediatr. 2015;27(3):303–7.
38. Long SS, Pickering LK, Charles G. Principles and practice of pediatric infectious diseases. Philadelphia: Elsevier; 2012. p. 454–62.
39. Trenchs V, Hernandez-Bou S, Bianchi C, Arnan M, Gene A, Luaces C. Blood cultures are not useful in the evaluation of children with uncomplicated superficial skin and soft tissue infections. Pediatr Infect Dis J. 2015;34(9):924–7.

Chapter 4
Fungal Infections in the Pediatric Age Group

Luluah Al-Mubarak, Colleen Cotton, and Sheila Fallon Friedlander

Abstract Cutaneous fungal infections occur in the pediatric age group and are a particular concern when they occur in premature or otherwise immunocompromised children. Clinical manifestations can result from infection with yeasts as well as dermatophytes. The most common fungal infection in healthy infants is Candida diaper dermatitis, which usually occurs as a secondary phenomenon following the development of contact dermatitis from the irritating effects of stool and urine. Candida paronychia from thumb-sucking may also occur in this age group. Older children are more likely to contract dermatophyte infections, sometimes transmitted from pets (e.g., Microsporum canis scalp or skin infections) or from other infected individuals (Trichophyton tonsurans). Adolescents are at higher risk for pityrosporum infections (commonly labeled with the misnomer tinea versicolor) and dermatophyte infections of the groin, feet, and nails. Systemic infection from any of the aforementioned infections does not occur in healthy, immunocompetent infants and children. Premature and immunocompromised individuals however are at risk for invasive infection with common pathogens such as Candida, pityrosporum, and opportunistic fungal pathogens such as Aspergillus. The increased incidence of immunosuppressed children, the use of immunosuppressive agents, and broad-spectrum anti-infective drugs make life-threatening infections from ubiquitous fungi a more common occurrence in children. A high index of suspicion for these disorders in at-risk populations, and early recognition of suspicious lesions is crucial to decrease associated morbidity and mortality. In this chapter, we will present several representative cases of fungal infections with potential for significant consequences in the pediatric population.

L. Al-Mubarak, MD
Department of Dermatology, Prince Sultan Military Medical City, Riyadh, Saudi Arabia

C. Cotton, MD
Division of Dermatology, Department of Medicine, University of Arizona, Tucson, AZ, USA

S.F. Friedlander, MD (✉)
Department of Dermatology and Pediatrics, University of California San Diego School of Medicine/Rady Children's Hospital, 8010 Frost Street, Suite 602, San Diego, CA 92123, USA
e-mail: poden@rchsd.org

© Springer International Publishing Switzerland 2016
M. Hogeling (ed.), *Case-Based Inpatient Pediatric Dermatology*,
DOI 10.1007/978-3-319-31569-0_4

Keywords Fungal infection • Pediatrics • Candida • Aspergillus • Tinea • Opportunistic fungal infection • Mucormycosis

Case 4.1

History

A 570 g female twin infant was born at the 25th week of gestation by Caesarian section with Apgar scores 7, 9, and 9. The pregnancy was complicated by maternal chorioamnionitis at the time of delivery. The infant was intubated, ventilated, and received surfactant because of respiratory distress syndrome. An umbilical catheter was placed in the first hours of life. Systemic antibiotic therapy was initiated with cefotaxime which was discontinued at day 7 when she was extubated. You are consulted for evaluation of non-healing cutaneous erosions present on the abdomen and left flank since birth. These were thought to be secondary to the trauma of childbirth; however, concern increased when they did not improve over time. Relevant history included prior maternal HSV labialis, quiescent at the time of birth. Twin B died at 2 days of age.

Physical Exam (Fig. 4.1)

Vitals: heart rate 153, blood pressure 46/24, O_2 sat 94%.

Laboratory Parameters

- Blood cultures: negative
- Placental pathology: no organisms noted. Fusion of placenta

Questions

1. What is your diagnosis?
2. What are the most likely causative organisms?
3. Would you like any additional tests?
4. What is your differential diagnosis?
5. What treatment would you consider?

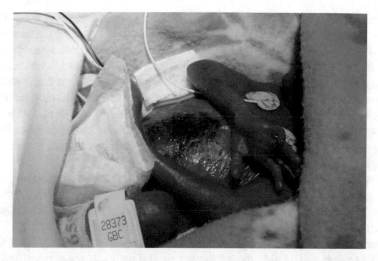

Fig. 4.1 A premature neonate with superficial adherent hemorrhagic dried crust on central mid-line abdomen with notable circinate sparing of umbilicus. Left flank exhibited re-epithelialized erosions

Answer

Cutaneous candidiasis.

Discussion

At birth, fetal skin is functionally incomplete and immature. Keratinization is not initiated until 22–24 weeks of gestation and continues over the first few weeks of life [1]. Premature infants have a high risk of developing dermatologic infections as a consequence of skin barrier immaturity. Opportunistic infections are an increasing concern in premature infants and neonates. Fungi are a particular concern if the patient has received prior and/or prolonged antibiotics. There are many factors that increase the risk of infection such as immunosuppression, intravenous catheters, iatrogenic skin trauma, broad-spectrum antibiotic use, and systemic corticosteroids [2].

Candida infections can cause benign, local mucocutaneous infections as well as invasive fatal systemic infections of any organ. Candida albicans accounts for the majority of Candida infections in neonates, but other species, including C. parapsilosis, C. tropicalis, and C. glabrata are also seen [3].

There are two main types of Candida infections in newborns—congenital candidiasis, which is acquired antenatally, and neonatal candidiasis, which is acquired during the perinatal or postnatal periods [4]. Many risk factors for candidiasis exist, which include but are not limited to premature infants, in particular those of very low birth weight (<1000 g) or less than 27 weeks gestation, the use of invasive devices and procedures (e.g., central venous catheters, mechanical ventilation), the use of broad-spectrum antibiotics, treatment with corticosteroids, prolonged use of parenteral nutrition, the presence of gastrointestinal pathology including congenital anomalies and necrotizing enterocolitis, hematopoietic disorders and neutropenia, the use of histamine type 2 receptor blockers, and the presence of hospital construction and renovation [1]. Patients are at risk not for only cutaneous infection but also for systemic disease, which may include pneumonia, meningitis, and sepsis [5].

Cutaneous Candida infection can have many presentations including papules, vesicles, pustules, ecchymosis, crusted lesions, and necrotic plaques. Premature infants and neonates who exhibit rapidly progressive erythema with erosions and desquamation are more likely to have systemic involvement (see Fig. 4.1).

In extremely low birth weight neonates, the invasive fungal dermatitis usually initially presents as Candida diaper dermatitis and then subsequently experience a rapidly progressive erosive dermatitis which can ultimately lead to a systemic infection. This emphasizes the importance of early diagnosis and monitoring of premature infants with suspected cutaneous fungal infections [6].

Most cases of cutaneous Candida infection are usually diagnosed by histopathology and culture [7]. Specimens obtained from patients should be sent for Gram stain, Tzanck staining, acid-fast bacilli (AFB), and potassium hydroxide (KOH)/PAS staining for completeness, as well as bacterial and mycobacterial culture [2]. Also, blood cultures are a necessary component of the evaluation of immunocompromised patients with fever. The differential diagnosis of erosions and crusts in neonates includes trauma, infections (Group B strep, Pseudomonas aeruginosa, Herpes simplex, Aspergillus, and Zygomycosis), and genetic disease (epidermolysis bullosa, Goltz syndrome) [2]. In the case of suspected systemic candidiasis, premature neonates require systemic antifungal therapy. For invasive Candida infection, intravenous amphotericin B is considered first-line therapy although combination therapy is recommended by some experts for protracted or severe cases [2]. Systemic fluconazole or itraconazole are alternative therapies.

Case 4.2

History

A 16-year-old female presented complaining of a red scaling rash on the hands for almost 6 months. She initially utilized a moderate potency topical corticosteroid but discontinued the treatment recently since it appeared to make the dermatitis worse.

Physical Exam (Fig. 4.2)

Questions

1. What is your diagnosis?
2. What are the most likely causative organisms?
3. Would you like any additional tests?
4. What is your differential diagnosis?
5. What treatment would you consider?

Answer

Majocchi's Granuloma.

Discussion

Tinea corporis is a dermatophytic infection of the skin which occurs mainly on the trunk and extremities and is usually restricted to the stratum corneum. Majocchi's granuloma is a deeper form of cutaneous fungal infection which was first described in 1883 by Domenico Majocchi [8]. It is a less common infection, sometimes

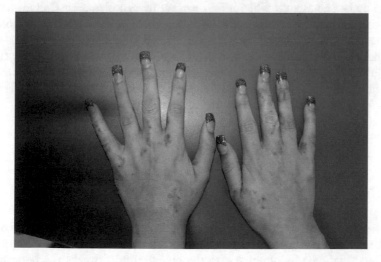

Fig. 4.2 A healthy teenage girl with multiple annular erythematous scaly plaques noted on bilateral dorsal hands

associated with depilation or the inappropriate use of high potency topical cortico-steroid therapy in an area of tinea corporis mistaken for eczema [9]. The pathogenesis of Majocchi's granuloma is thought to result from a nodular perifolliculitis with subsequent formation of a foreign body granuloma, resulting from infection of the dermis and subcutaneous tissue by dermatophytes. Dermatophyte infection in Majocchi's granuloma causes rupture of the hair follicle infundibulum which leads to dermal and subcutaneous tissue inflammation, resulting in the typical clinical finding of chronic erythematous and indurated plaques [10]. In immunocompetent patients and as seen in our case (see Fig. 4.2). Trichophyton rubrum is the most common dermatophyte isolated, but other fungi have been reported including Trichophyton mentagrophytes, Trichophyton violaceum, and Epidermophyton floccosum [9, 11]. Follicular invasion in Majocchi's granuloma is usually endothrix in nature. An endo-ectothrix mosaic pattern can also be detected. There are two clinical forms of Majocchi's granuloma [12]. The first or superficial type is formed by granulomatous inflammation limited to the perifollicular area [12]. It usually affects a healthy individual after localized trauma, chronic use of topical corticosteroid use, or chronic foot dermatophyte colonization. It can be seen in young women who repeatedly shave their legs or after chronic use of corticosteroid treatment. The second, or deeper form, is usually seen in immunocompromised patients and is characterized by a subcutaneous granulomatous response and neutrophilic dermal abscesses [10]. Trauma is also thought to be an initiating factor in some of the deeper cases. Cell-mediated immune depression and a blunted inflammatory response, leading to inhibition of response to the dermatophyte, may contribute to progression of the disease. Differential diagnosis of Majocchi's granuloma includes atopic dermatitis, subcutaneous lupus, and other deep fungal infections and granulomatous disorders.

The diagnosis is confirmed through direct mycological examination, culture, and/or histopathology. On histopathological examination, one can see giant cell and foreign body granulomas which often contain hyphal elements. Culture or KOH evaluation is important; however, the histopathological as well as mycological examination may not reveal fungal elements. Specific fungal stains, such as the periodic acid–Schiff stain or Gomori methenamine-silver, may be necessary to visualize fungal elements in tissues. Systemic antifungals, such as azole antifungals, griseofulvin and terbinafine, are the mainstays of therapy. Treatment should be continued for at least 4–8 weeks, and until all lesions have cleared.

Case 4.3

History

A 3-year-old female presented to the hospital with fever, coryza, diarrhea, and new mouth ulcers. A complete blood count (CBC) revealed a profound pancytopenia with blasts, and she was admitted to the hospital for further workup. A bone marrow biopsy confirmed the diagnosis of acute pre B-cell lymphoblastic leukemia. Broad-spectrum antibiotic therapy (cefepime and meropenem) was initiated.

Six days after admission, shortly after initiation of her chemotherapy, the patient develops erythematous papules at the site of her intravenous catheter (IV). You are consulted because over the course of 3 days, the papules have become increasingly tender, and dark vesicles with surrounding erythema have developed at the site. Today, the patient also developed a fever, after being afebrile for several days. Her initial blood cultures obtained at admission were negative.

Physical Exam (Fig. 4.3)

Laboratory Parameters

- White blood count: 1.0 (4.0–10.5 K/μL)
  - Segmented neutrophils: 5 (45–70 %)
  - Lymphocytes: 94 (15–50 %)
  - Monocytes: 1 (2–12 %)

- Hemoglobin: 8.0 (12.5–16.1 g/dL)
- Platelets: 53 (140–440 K/μL)
- AST: 133 (15–40 U/L)
- ALT: 219 (10–45 U/L)
- Blood cultures from 6 days prior showed no growth
- Computed tomography (CT) of the chest, abdomen, and pelvis demonstrates hepatomegaly, but is otherwise unremarkable
- Magnetic resonance imaging (MRI) of the right wrist demonstrates mild edema and soft-tissue inflammation at the radial aspect of the wrist. Diffuse abnormal signal in the bone marrow of the hand, wrist, and arm likely represents leukemic infiltration

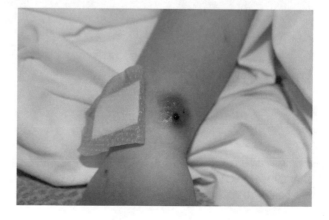

Fig. 4.3 Physical examination reveals three erythematous, indurated violaceous papules and nodules with central necrosis on the distal right forearm/wrist

Fig. 4.4 H&E stain showing necrosis and fungal hyphal elements invading into the subcutaneous fat. *White arrow*: hyphae are broad, infrequently septate, and of irregular width

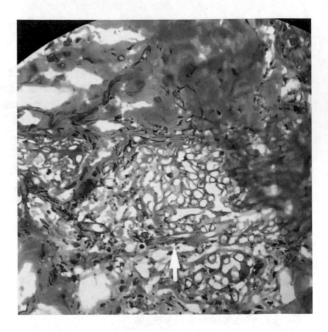

- 4 mm punch biopsy of the right wrist demonstrates epidermal necrosis and ulceration with abundant fungal elements extending to the deep dermis and subcutaneous fat with foci of intravascular invasion (Fig. 4.4)

Questions

1. What is your diagnosis?
2. What are the most likely causative organisms?
3. Would you like any additional imaging or tests?
4. What treatment would you consider?

Answer

Primary Cutaneous Mucormycosis.

Discussion

Primary cutaneous fungal infections are an important diagnostic consideration in immunocompromised patients. These infections occur through damage to the epidermis that then facilitates fungal entry into the skin and subcutaneous tissue.

The typical presentation is that of paronychia in the setting of onychomycosis or cellulitis at the site of an IV [13]. Lesions at sites of trauma are usually a red or purpuric plaque containing papules, pustules, or vesicles with subsequent central necrosis. The most common causative agents include Aspergillus, Candida, and Fusarium species, as well as zygomycetes like Mucor and Rhizopus [14]. Aspergillus and Rhizopus are the classic culprits in IV and arm board lesions [13]. The differential diagnosis includes bacterial infection, particularly ecthyma gangrenosum, as well as leukemia cutis. Cutaneous fungal infections can appear identical to bacterial paronychia and cellulitis, but may sometimes be differentiated by the presence of purpura or an eschar. Biopsy can be used to distinguish these different entities.

The incidence of opportunistic fungal infection is highest in children with hematologic malignancies, such as acute lymphocytic and myelogenous leukemia, as well as those undergoing allogeneic hematopoietic stem cell transplants [15]. The most predictive risk factor is the presence of prolonged, severe neutropenia. Other risk factors include maceration from tape or occlusive dressings, vascular and urinary catheters, broad-spectrum antibiotics, disruption of the mucosal surface secondary to trauma or chemotherapy, and graft versus host disease [13]. Diabetes mellitus and systemic immunosuppression also increase risk, though not to the same degree.

Early diagnosis and initiation of appropriate antifungal treatment are crucial [16]. Tissue biopsy with histology and culture should be performed for any suspicious lesions. Often blood and tissue cultures fail to demonstrate the organism, making histology the best option in order to rapidly identify the etiology, initiate early treatment and reduce mortality. Parental or child apprehension regarding the procedure should not delay biopsy, and conscious sedation may be helpful if it can be arranged in a timely fashion [17]. Demonstration of fungal organisms invading tissue is ideal, though not always seen on pathology. The morphology of observed fungal elements can be used to identify the likely group of species and guide treatment. As many of the causative organisms are common in the environment, positive culture alone is not proof of infection, though repeat cultures that are positive specifically for the same organism can be strongly suggestive. A "deep slide prep" may also be performed by smearing a glass slide with only the deep portion of a specimen.

Many of these fungal pathogens have a propensity for angioinvasion. The potential for dissemination is quite high, and these infections demonstrate a 30–80 % mortality rate depending on the organism and referenced study [13, 18]. Mucormycosis, the offending pathogen in this case, has an especially high risk of dissemination as compared to Aspergillus or other fungi [18]. Additional imaging is required to evaluate deep tissue infection for secondary systemic disease, particularly of the lungs, GI tract, and underlying bone and musculature. Although blood cultures are often negative, they should still be followed, especially if the patient remains febrile.

Treatment

As stated above, prompt treatment with a systemic antifungal is key to reducing morbidity and mortality. Consultation with the Infectious Disease service should be initiated early to tailor antifungal therapy to the suspected organism based on histology and/or culture [19]. Systemic antifungal options include amphotericin B, caspofungin, micafungin, fluconazole, voriconazole, posaconazole, and itraconazole. Different fungal organisms respond to each of these medications with varying efficacy. Infected patients who are neutropenic should receive inpatient antifungal treatment until their neutropenia resolves [13]. In this case, the patient underwent prompt surgical debridement and was treated with several months of amphotericin B.

For primary skin disease, debridement is thought to be helpful. Fungal invasion may extend well beyond the borders of the clinically apparent lesion. Recommendations differ as to whether patients should undergo urgent debridement upon diagnosis, or if they should be pretreated with systemic antifungals for several days prior to surgery [13, 18, 19]. Surgical excision of affected tissue is especially important with Mucormycosis, given a lack of reliable systemic therapies. Systemic antifungal treatment should continue for at least 2–3 weeks after debridement to avoid recurrence. Total duration should be determined based on clinical signs, symptoms, and status of underlying immunocompromised [19].

Case 4.4

History

A 14-year-old male was admitted for management of newly diagnosed acute myelogenous leukemia (AML). On the day following completion of a 2-week course of intrathecal and systemic induction chemotherapy, the patient developed new skin lesions on the buttocks and bilateral thighs. The patient was reportedly scratching one of these lesions and it bled earlier in the day. The lesions seem to be spreading. He is febrile this morning for the first time in several days, and has had multiple negative blood cultures. Patient denies any sinus tenderness or shortness of breath, though he has had a light cough for the last 2 days. Current medications include acyclovir for herpes simplex virus (HSV) prophylaxis, trimethoprim-sulfamethoxazole for Pneumocystis prophylaxis, and cefepime for neutropenic fever.

Physical Exam (Figs. 4.5 and 4.6)

Laboratory Parameters

- White blood count: 0.5 (4.0–10.5 K/μL)

  - Segmented neutrophils: 22 (45–70 %)
  - Lymphocytes: 30 (15–50 %)
  - Blasts: 40 (0–0 %)

Fig. 4.5 Physical examination reveals diffuse violaceous hyperpigmentation over the buttocks with retiform purpura, as well as discrete violaceous papules and plaques on the bilateral lower extremities

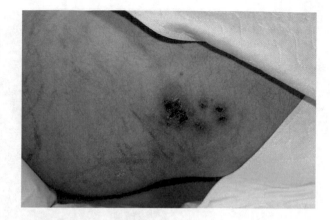

Fig. 4.6 Close-up of the right posterior thigh, showing multiple violaceous papules coalescing into a 7 cm × 4 cm plaque with central necrosis and surrounding erythema. This plaque was tender to touch

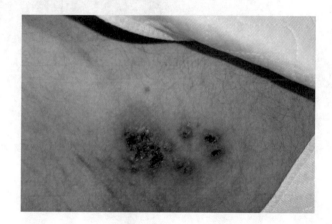

- Hemoglobin: 8.1 (12.5–16.1 g/dL)
- Platelets: 15 (140–440 K/μL)
- AST: 137 (15–40 U/L)
- ALT: 225 (10–45 U/L)
- Blood cultures from 7, 5, and 4 days prior show no growth
- CT scan of chest: punctate nodular opacities throughout the right lung with a "tree-in-bud" appearance
- Imaging of sinuses, abdomen, and pelvis within normal limits
- 4 mm punch biopsy of right thigh plaque shows ulcerated skin with invasion of fungal hyphal elements of irregular width and right-angle branching extending to the mid-dermis (Fig. 4.7)

Fig. 4.7 H&E stain showing right-angle branching morphology of broad, infrequently septate morphology of hyphae. *Black arrow*: right-angle branching; *white arrows*: additional invasive hyphae

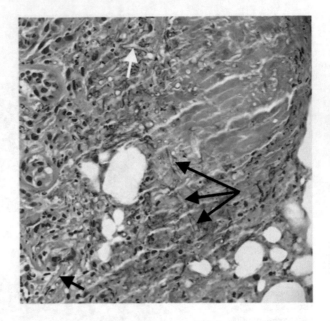

Questions

1. What is your differential diagnosis?
2. What are the most likely causative organisms?
3. In what ways is this case similar to Case 4.3? In what ways does it differ?

Answer

Disseminated systemic Zygomycosis: Rhizopus.

Discussion

Opportunistic systemic fungal infections are an important cause of morbidity and mortality in immunocompromised patients, though they occasionally can be seen in immunocompetent patients as well [13]. Not all opportunistic fungi disseminate to the skin, so an absence of skin lesions does not preclude systemic fungal infection. Other causes of neutropenic fever should be included in the differential diagnosis, including bacterial sepsis, endocarditis, and tumor lysis syndrome. Blood cultures, histology, electrolytes, and lactate dehydrogenase (LDH) levels can help to distinguish these diseases. It is important to remember that the presence of one diagnosis (e.g., positive bacterial blood culture) does not preclude the others, and so a full work-up should always be completed.

The most likely causative organisms that the dermatologist will encounter are Fusarium, Aspergillus, and Candida, though zygomycetes, Cryptococcus, and Trichosporon beigelii may rarely be seen [13]. Common initial sites of infection include the GI tract (Candida in particular), sinuses, lungs, primary skin lesions, and infected catheters. Cutaneous manifestations of systemic disease may present as tender, erythematous macules or plaques that progress to develop areas of necrosis and/or vesiculation. Fusarium infections tend to have more numerous lesions favoring the extremities over the trunk, whereas Aspergillus lesions tend to be larger and fewer in numbers [20]. Skin lesions of Candida fungemia tend to be pink dermal papules that may occasionally become purpuric but not typically necrotic.

The major differentiator between primary and secondary cutaneous disease is the number of lesions. Solitary lesions at a site of trauma will most likely be primary, whereas the presence of multiple lesions is much more suggestive of secondary disease. In this case, identifying the initial source of fungemia is critical for initiation of appropriate treatment. Imaging of the sinuses and lungs is required. Early in disease, fungal sinusitis may not be evident on CT, making MRI potentially superior [21]. Fungal pneumonia may present with a "tree-in-bud" appearance on high-resolution CT scan, representing infectious bronchiolitis, or "halo" or "air-crescent" signs representing aspergillosis. In this case, the initial source of disease was a Rhizopus pneumonia.

Early tissue biopsy for histology and culture is crucial for making the diagnosis and directing treatment. Microscopic appearance of fungal elements can and should guide choice of antifungal therapy [19]. Broad, irregularly shaped, non-septate hyphae with 90°-branching suggests zygomycosis (e.g., Mucor, Rhizopus), while septate hyphae branching at a 45° angle is consistent with Aspergillus and Fusarium species. Cryptococcus can be identified as yeast-like organisms with a characteristic halo representing a capsule.

In many cases, blood cultures in patients with systemic fungal infections will be negative [22]. The exception is with disseminated Fusarium, though even with this organism, the skin lesions may predate positive blood cultures by several days [20]. There are two major serologic fungal antigens that can be used in the diagnosis and monitoring of systemic fungal infection. Galactomannan is a polysaccharide from the Aspergillus cell wall and may be used to detect disease early and follow response to treatment. However, its use is limited by a high false-positive rate in pediatric patients and bone marrow transplant patients, likely due in part to interfering antibiotics like piperacillin/tazobactam and amoxicillin [22]. The other major antigen is 1,3-beta-D-glucan, a cell wall component of several pathogenic fungi. This assay is limited by lack of data in the pediatric population, a high rate of false-positives in patients with hematologic malignancies, and a high baseline concentration in immunocompetent uninfected children [22]. Both antigens by definition will miss some causes of disseminated fungal infections, including Mucor, Rhizopus, and Cryptococcus. Real-time polymerase chain reaction (PCR) studies of whole blood show promise, but are not standardized [22].

Treatment

Treatment for systemic opportunistic fungal infection is similar to treatment previously discussed for primary cutaneous disease [13, 19]. Choice of systemic antifungal should be based on the responsible pathogen. Treatment courses usually last several months and should continue at least until complete clinical remission is achieved. Surgical debridement may be required for skin lesions that are larger or more necrotic. Patients with sinusitis require surgery in addition to systemic antifungals for cure. In this case, the patient was treated empirically with voriconazole, and then quickly switched to posaconazole and amphotericin B once the fungus was identified as Rhizopus. Repeated debridement of the large thigh plaque was required, ultimately necessitating a Wound-Vac, and his pneumonia persisted for 2 months. Systemic treatment was required for 4 months.

The question of chemoprophylaxis has arisen to help prevent the high morbidity and mortality associated with opportunistic fungal infections. There is a need for standardized regimens in high-risk patient groups, such as those with hematologic malignancies and those undergoing bone marrow transplant. A few courses of therapy have been proposed, and in general posaconazole and voriconazole are the two major drugs of choice [19, 23]. However, the local epidemiology must be considered, and so a "one-size-fits-all" solution is not entirely practical [19]. In patients who have previously contracted and survived an opportunistic fungal infection, secondary chemoprophylaxis is often employed, though there is no strong evidence to support this practice [19, 23].

Conflict of Interest Dr. Friedlander has conducted research on topical antifungal lacquers for Valeant Pharmaceuticals and served as a consultant for Sandoz Pharmaceuticals.

References

1. Smolinski KN, Shah SS, Honig PJ, Yan AC. Neonatal cutaneous fungal infections. Curr Opin Pediatr. 2005;17(4):486–93.
2. Hook KP, Eichenfield LF. Approach to the neonate with ecchymoses and crusts. Dermatol Ther. 2011;24(2):240–8.
3. Levy I, Rubin LG, Vasishtha S, et al. Emergence of Candida parapsilosis as the predominant species causing candidemia in children. Clin Infect Dis. 1998;26:1086–8.
4. Rowen JL. Mucocutaneous candidiasis. Semin Perinatol. 2003;27:406–13.
5. Diana A, Epiney M, Ecoffey M, Pfister RE. 'White dots on the placenta and red dots on the baby': congenital cutaneous candidiasis—a rare disease of the neonate. Acta Paediatr. 2004;93:996–9.
6. Passeron T, Desruelles F, Gari-Toussaint M, et al. Invasive fungal dermatitis in a 770 gram neonate. Pediatr Dermatol. 2004;21:260–1.
7. Roilides E, Zaoutis TE, Walsh TJ. Invasive zygomycosis in neonates and children. Clin Microbiol Infect. 2009;15 Suppl 5:50–4.
8. Kanaan IC, Santos TB, Kac BK, Souza AM, Cerqueira AM. Majocchi's granuloma—case report. An Bras Dermatol. 2015;90(2):251–3.

9. Bressan AL, Silva RS, Fonseca JC, de Alves MF. Majocchi's granuloma. An Bras Dermatol. 2011;86:797–8.
10. Molina-Leyva A, Perez-Parra S, Garcia-Garcia F. Case for diagnosis. An Bras Dermatol. 2014;89(5):839–40.
11. Chen HH, Chiu HC. Facial Majocchi's granuloma caused by Trichophyton tonsurans in an immunocompetent patient. Acta Derm Venereol. 2003;83:65–6.
12. Kim JE, Won CH, Chang S, Lee MW, Choi JH, Moon KC. Majocchi's granuloma mimicking Kaposi sarcoma in a heart transplant patient. J Dermatol. 2011;38:927–9.
13. Mays SR, Bogle MA, Bodey GP. Cutaneous fungal infections in the oncology patient: recognition and management. Am J Clin Dermatol. 2006;7(1):31–43.
14. Grossman ME. Cutaneous manifestations of infection in the immunocompromised host. Baltimore: Williams & Wilkins; 1995. p. 188.
15. Brown AE. Overview of fungal infections in cancer patients. Semin Oncol. 1990;17(3 Suppl 6):2–5.
16. Dekio F, Bhatti TR, Zhang SX, Sullivan KV. Positive impact of fungal histopathology on immunocompromised pediatric patients with histology-proven invasive fungal infection. Am J Clin Pathol. 2015;144(1):61–7.
17. Sirignano S, Blake P, Turrentine JE, Dominguez AR. Primary cutaneous zygomycosis secondary to minor trauma in an immunocompromised pediatric patient: a case report. Dermatol Online J. 2014;15:20(6).
18. Roden MM, et al. Epidemiology and outcome of zygomycosis: a review of 929 reported cases. Clin Infect Dis. 2005;41(5):634–53.
19. Groll AH, et al. Fourth European Conference on Infections in Leukaemia (ECIL-4): guidelines for diagnosis, prevention, and treatment of invasive fungal diseases in paediatric patients with cancer or allogeneic haemopoietic stem-cell transplantation. Lancet Oncol. 2014;15(8):e327–40.
20. Bodey GP, et al. Skin lesions associated with Fusarium infection. J Am Acad Dermatol. 2002;47(5):659–66.
21. Howells RC, Ramadan HH. Usefulness of computed tomography and magnetic resonance in fulminant invasive fungal rhinosinusitis. Am J Rhinol. 2001;15(4):255–61.
22. Oz Y, Kiraz N. Diagnostic methods for fungal infections in pediatric patients: microbiological, serological and molecular methods. Expert Rev Anti Infect Ther. 2011;9(3):289–98.
23. Tragiannidis A, Dokos C, Lehrnbecher T, Groll AH. Antifungal chemoprophylaxis in children and adolescents with haematological malignancies and following allogeneic haematopoietic stem cell transplantation: review of the literature and options for clinical practice. Drugs. 2012;72(5):685–704.

Chapter 5
Drug Eruptions and Hypersensitivity Syndromes

Nicole N. Harter and Minnelly Luu

Abstract Drug eruptions and hypersensitivity reactions are commonly encountered diagnoses in inpatient pediatric dermatology and can range from simple cutaneous eruptions to severe, life-threatening systemic reactions. Although etiology varies by diagnosis, these reactions are most often triggered by medication exposure and/or infectious agents. In this chapter, we review the presentation, pathogenesis, diagnosis, and management of the most common and/or severe drug and hypersensitivity reactions with emphasis on features distinct in the pediatric population. Case discussions include acute urticaria, urticaria multiforme, erythema multiforme, Stevens–Johnson syndrome, toxic epidermal necrolysis, morbilliform drug eruption, drug reaction with eosinophilia and systemic symptoms, acute generalized exanthematous pustulosis, and erythema nodosum. Dermatologists, pediatricians, and inpatient pediatric providers should be familiar with the presentation and differential diagnoses of these conditions and their unique characteristics in children.

Keywords Pediatric • Children • Hypersensitivity • Drug eruption • Drug reaction • Acute urticaria • Urticaria multiforme • Stevens–Johnson Syndrome (SJS) • Toxic epidermal necrolysis (TEN) • Morbilliform • Drug reaction with eosinophilia and systemic symptoms (DRESS) • Acute generalized exanthematous pustulosis (AGEP) • Erythema nodosum (EN)

N.N. Harter, BS, MD • M. Luu, MD (✉)
Department of Dermatology, Children's Hospital Los Angeles, Keck School of Medicine of USC, 4640 Sunset Blvd., Mailstop 144, Los Angeles, CA, USA
e-mail: mluu@chla.usc.edu

© Springer International Publishing Switzerland 2016
M. Hogeling (ed.), *Case-Based Inpatient Pediatric Dermatology*,
DOI 10.1007/978-3-319-31569-0_5

Abbreviations

AGEP	Acute generalized exanthematous pustulosis
ALT	Amino alanine transferase
ANA	Anti-nuclear antibody
ASO	Anti-streptolysin O
AST	Aspartate amino transferase
BSA	Body surface area
CBC	Complete blood count
CMP	Complete metabolic panel
Cr	Creatinine
CRP	C-reactive protein
CMV	Cytomegalovirus
DIF	Direct immunofluorescence
DIHS	Drug-induced hypersensitivity syndrome
DNAse B	Deoxyribonuclease B
DRESS	Drug reaction with eosinophilia and systemic symptoms
EBV	Epstein–Barr virus
EKG	Electrocardiogram
EM	Erythema multiforme
EN	Erythema nodosum
ENT	Ear-nose-and-throat
ESR	Erythrocyte sedimentation rate
EN	Erythema nodosum
Gamma GT	Gamma glutamyl transpeptidase
G-CSF	Granulocyte colony-stimulating factor
H	High
Hct	Hematocrit
HIV	Human immunodeficiency virus
Hgb	Hemoglobin
HHV-6	Human herpes virus-6
HLA	Human leukocyte antigen
HSV	Herpes simplex virus
IIF	Indirect immunofluorescence
IL-5	Interleukin-5
IV	Intravenous
IVIG	Intravenous immunoglobulin
LFT	Liver function test
L	Low
N	Normal
NSAID	Non-steroidal anti-inflammatory drug
NUD	Neutrophilic urticarial dermatosis
OTC	Over-the-counter
PO	Per Os

Plt	Platelet
SJS	Stevens–Johnson syndrome
SSSS	Staphylococcal scalded skin syndrome
TEN	Toxic epidermal necrolysis
TNF-α	Tumor necrosis factor-alpha
WBC	White blood cells
WNL	Within normal limits

Case 5.1

History

A 17-year-old previously healthy male presented to the emergency department with a diffuse rash that began 5 days prior to admission, first appearing on the arm and subsequently spreading to involve his entire trunk as well as arms and legs. He and his parents are not sure whether lesions are transient because they are everywhere. He complains of severe pruritus, for which he has applied diphenhydramine topical cream without relief. He had a mild episode of coughing and congestion approximately 1 week ago, and he denies shortness of breath, wheezing, facial swelling, lip swelling, or joint pains. Medication history is negative.

Physical Examination (Fig. 5.1)

Laboratory

- Normal CBC with differential, CMP, ESR, and CRP

Questions

1. What features of the physical examination and history might be important in determining the diagnosis?
2. What is the differential diagnosis for this patient?
3. What is the management for this patient?

Fig. 5.1 Annular and
gyrate, edematous,
pink-red papules and
plaques on trunk, upper
extremities, lower
extremities.
Dermatographism is
present. A discrete lesion is
marked with a pen and
shows significant
improvement by the next
day. Photo courtesy of
Alexandra Haden, M.D.

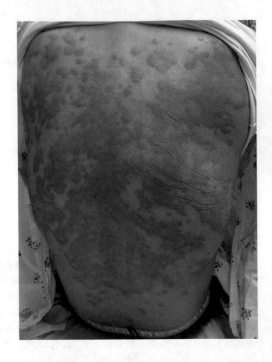

Answer

Acute urticaria is characterized by sudden appearance of evanescent, edematous, pale-pink, intensely pruritic wheals. The eruption is very common, occurring at some point in 15–20 % of the general population and in 2.1–6.7 % of children [1–3]. Urticaria may be mediated by immunologic or non-immunologic pathways [4]. Immunologic urticaria is a type I immediate hypersensitivity reaction characterized by binding of IgE to the surface of mast cells. This results in release of histamine and vasoactive cytokines, causing increased capillary permeability and extravasation of fluid which results in edematous papules and plaques [3, 5]. Non-immunologic urticaria occurs when antigens directly trigger mast cell degranulation, seen with NSAIDs, aspirin, and opiates [2, 4]. By definition, acute urticaria lasts less than 6 weeks in duration, distinguishing it from chronic urticaria [1, 3].

Clinically, urticaria can take on multiple morphologies, such as formation of annular, polycyclic, gyrate, or figurate patterns, and may range in size from 1 mm to several centimeters as lesions coalesce into larger plaques. Individual wheals resolve in less than 24 h, a clinical feature that is helpful diagnostically, while the patient may continue to develop lesions in new areas [1, 3]. Urticaria may be isolated to one region or develop diffusely over the body. In very young children, bullae may develop within the center of the wheal [2]. Pruritus may not always be a primary complaint in pediatric urticaria, though certain features are reported with greater frequency. In a prospective study evaluating acute urticaria in infancy and early childhood 50 % of patients had associated angioedema and 60 % presented with ecchymotic lesions [6, 7]. In this study, a cause for acute urticaria was identified in 92 % of cases; however, this number varies greatly in the literature, with reports from 21 to 90 % [3, 6].

In the pediatric population, the most common etiology of acute urticaria is infection, predominately viral, as in this case, however there have been associations with a multitude of infectious agents [1–3, 6, 7]. Food and medication are also frequent triggers, more often seen in older children and teenagers, with drugs causing up to 10 % of these eruptions [2]. The most commonly implicated medications include antimicrobials, notably beta-lactams (penicillins, cephalosporins), macrolides, sulfonamides, and tetracyclines as well as anticonvulsants, aspirin, NSAIDs, monoclonal antibodies, opioids, and radiocontrast media [2, 8]. Food allergy is notably infrequently cited as a cause of acute urticaria in the literature [3, 9]. In a multicenter study evaluating cutaneous adverse drug reactions in children, urticaria and angioedema were the most common adverse events, affecting 51.6 % of the study population, with primary triggers including antimicrobials, analgesics, antiinflammatories, and antipyretics [10]. There are also reports of urticaria occurring secondary to vaccine administration [11].

Depending on clinical morphology, the differential diagnosis may include erythema multiforme, urticaria multiforme, or serum-sickness like reaction. If wheals remain fixed beyond 24 h, urticarial vasculitis should be considered in the differential diagnosis [2, 12]. Other vasculitides, such as Henoch–Schönlein purpura and acute hemorrhagic edema of infancy, may also occasionally enter into the differential, especially during their early stages. If the child is febrile or displays vital sign or laboratory abnormalities, other systemic etiologies should be considered, including cryopyrin-associated periodic syndromes and systemic-onset juvenile idiopathic arthritis [12]. Papular urticaria may be considered, which is specific to the pediatric population and characterized by pruritic, edematous papules that are secondary to arthropod assault [1].

As the clinical presentation is usually quite classic, laboratory investigation or skin biopsy are rarely required for diagnosis and should only be considered in the patient with atypical presentations, if the patient is otherwise systemically ill, or if urticaria persists for greater than 24 h to evaluate for urticarial vasculitis [13]. Histopathology of acute urticaria demonstrates vascular dilation, edema, and perivascular inflammatory infiltrate of lymphocytes, eosinophils, and neutrophils [5, 7]. Blood eosinophils may be elevated as well [7]. Urticarial lesions of auto-inflammatory syndromes such as cryopyrin-associated periodic syndromes show a deeper perivascular and perieccrine neutrophilic infiltrate with notably rare eosinophils and the absence of dermal edema, for which the term neutrophilic urticarial dermatosis (NUD) has been proposed [12, 14]. NUD has also been associated with adult-onset Still disease.

Treatment

Treatment of acute urticaria involves removing or avoiding the trigger, along with symptomatic care. This includes sedating, first-generation H1 antihistamines (hydroxyzine, diphenhydramine) in conjunction with non-sedating, second-generation H1 antihistamines (cetirizine, loratidine, fexofenadine) [1]. Notably, sedating antihistamines may cause paradoxical excitation in infants, while non-sedating preparations may be titrated up to fourfold the doses used in the treatment of allergic rhinitis, if necessary [2, 4, 7, 9]. H2 antihistamines may also be added (ranitidine, cimetidine) for recalcitrant or severe cases [1]. For optimum control, treatment should be continued for several weeks beyond clearance of urticaria [2]. In refractory cases, short courses of oral corticosteroids may be given [1].

Case 5.2

History

A 15-month-old otherwise healthy male presented to the emergency department due to a rash for 3 days. Ten days prior he developed fever, rhinorrhea, and cough. Subsequently, 3 days prior to presentation, he developed "hives" on his trunk, which progressed to larger "welts" over the next few days. The rash appears to be itchy. Two days ago he developed swelling of the hands and feet, and this morning his mother noted facial swelling, which prompted her to seek urgent care.

Review of systems is significant only for mildly decreased appetite and rhinorrhea. He does not have fever, lethargy, shortness of breath, wheezing, cough, diarrhea, vomiting, or difficulty ambulating. His mother reports that he is overall active and playful.

Physical Examination (Fig. 5.2)

Laboratory

• Normal CBC with differential and complete metabolic panel

Questions

1. What features of the physical examination and history might be important in determining the diagnosis?
2. What is the differential diagnosis?

Fig. 5.2 Large and confluent, as well as smaller and discrete, annular, edematous pink-red plaques with central clearing and gray-dusky discoloration involving the scalp, face, back, chest, abdomen, arms, legs, and dorsum of the hands and feet. Face, hands, and feet are edematous. There is 3+ dermatographism. Oral mucosa and conjunctiva are clear. Joints do not appear swollen

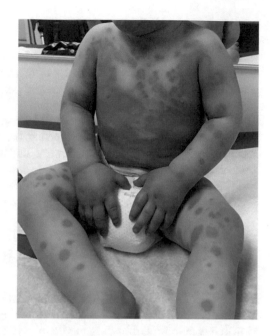

Answer

Urticaria multiforme is a benign, self-limited, cutaneous hypersensitivity reaction presenting in young children from several months to several years of age often occurring 1–3 days after a viral illness [6, 12]. It is considered a subtype of acute urticaria; however, the cutaneous presentation is unique and distinguished by characteristic arcuate, polycyclic, and annular urticarial plaques with dusky or ecchymotic centers [12, 15]. This annular presentation with dusky central clearing is often confused with erythema multiforme (EM), thus giving rise to its namesake [7].

Diagnostic criteria for this eruption have been proposed and include annular or polycyclic lesions with transient ecchymotic skin changes, individual lesions lasting <24–36 h, angioedema or acral edema, dermatographism, moderately elevated acute phase reactants, and positive response to antihistamines [7, 12, 16]. Patients may have associated fever and report symptoms of antecedent or concomitant viral illness [16].

The pathogenesis of urticaria multiforme overlaps with that of urticaria as an allergic hypersensitivity reaction that may be IgE dependent or independent. In one study, 50 % of children <3 years of age presenting with urticaria demonstrated a pattern consistent with urticaria multiforme [6]. Angioedema is often associated and has been described 60–72 % cases [6, 16, 17]. Antecedent respiratory viral and gastrointestinal viral and bacterial infections are commonly reported; however, this is often confounded by recent or concomitant antibiotic use, reported in 44 % of patients [16]. Urticaria multiforme has also been described after vaccine administration [12, 16, 17].

Laboratory analysis for infectious etiology is not recommended as the work-up often fails to provide clinically significant information. The diagnosis is made clinically from thorough history and physical exam, and therefore, skin biopsy is usually unnecessary. Histopathology of urticaria multiforme is not distinct from acute urticaria, showing dermal edema and perivascular infiltrate with eosinophils [12, 17].

The differential diagnosis includes EM; however, there are no true target lesions, bullae, epidermal sloughing, or mucous membrane involvement [16]. Serum-sickness like reaction, urticarial vasculitis, and acute hemorrhagic edema of infancy may also be considered; however, skin lesions are fixed in these entities. Patients with serum sickness-like reaction have arthralgias, as opposed to swelling of the hands and feet seen with urticarial multiforme [12, 17].

Treatment

Treatment of urticaria multiforme is supportive with sedating and non-sedating H1 and H2 anti-histamines, along with antipyretics for fever, and discontinuation of any potential offending medication [12]. Topical corticosteroids, pramoxine, or preparations containing colloidal oatmeal or menthol may be used to alleviate pruritus. Short-course systemic corticosteroids should be reserved for refractory cases only, with judicious use when infectious etiology is suspected [16, 17].

Case 5.3

History

A 12-year-old female with history of allergic rhinitis was admitted for evaluation of a rash, which began 4 days prior to admission. Two weeks prior to admission, patient developed fever, sore throat, and cough. She presented to her primary care provider, who prescribed cephalexin. One day after starting cephalexin, she developed lesions on her face, which progressed over the next several days. Cephalexin was discontinued, but the rash continued to worsen, prompting evaluation in the emergency department and admission.

Her review of systems is significant for cough, which is overall improving. She denies sore throat, dysphagia, photophobia, shortness of breath, chest pain, abdominal pain, vomiting, diarrhea, dysuria, or rectal pain. She denies sick contacts, history of cold sores, or history of allergy to medications. There are no family members with known cold sores.

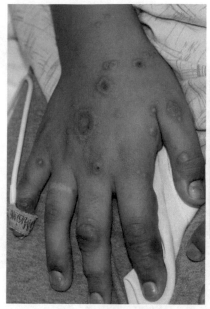
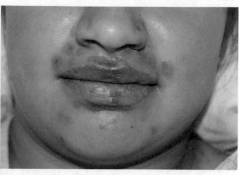

Fig. 5.3 Multiple round papules and plaques with erythematous periphery, edematous middle zone, and central vesicle with widespread distribution including the face, neck, abdomen, arms, hands, palms, thighs, legs, and feet. In many lesions, there is central erosion with hemorrhagic crusting rather than a vesicle. Areas of confluence are noted on the neck and arms. Vermillion lips are involved, but oral cavity and conjunctivae are intact. Anogenital examination reveals similar lesions on the mons pubis, buttocks, and gluteal cleft

Physical Examination (Fig. 5.3)

Laboratory

- Urinalysis negative
- Chest X-ray unremarkable
- Mycoplasma Pneumoniae IgM 1140 (H, >950 positive), IgG 1.94 (H, >1.1 positive)
- Lesional HSV PCR Negative

Questions

1. What are the pathognomonic morphologic features of this condition?
2. What are the most common triggers of this condition?

Answer

Erythema multiforme (EM) is an acute, self-limited mucocutaneous eruption characterized by distinct targetoid lesions on the skin. EM is most common in young-adults, with up to 20 % of cases occurring in children [2, 18, 19]. EM is considered a cell-mediated immune reaction to an intracellular antigen, which leads to local tissue damage [20, 21]. Greater than 90 % of cases occur secondary to infection, most commonly herpes simplex virus (HSV) and *Mycoplasma pneumoniae*; however, numerous infectious agents have been cited as triggers [22]. Medications have previously been implicated in <10 % of cases although a recent large-scale study performed in a pediatric tertiary care facility found 46 % of cases of non-bullous EM were associated with drugs, with this association being greatest in the youngest patients [23]. The most common offending agents include NSAIDs, penicillin, sulfonamides, antiepileptics, and other antibiotics [23, 24]. Reports have also cited EM occurring subsequent to vaccine administration [11, 21, 25].

EM ranges from a relatively mild cutaneous disease (EM minor) to a severe eruption with significant involvement of more than one mucosal surface (EM major) [18]. Previously EM was considered on a continuum with Stevens–Johnson Syndrome (SJS) and Toxic Epidermal Necrolysis (TEN), however EM is now generally regarded as a separate entity [21, 24]. It is distinguished from SJS/TEN by the presence of typical target lesions, inciting infectious stimulus, and more favorable prognosis with limited systemic symptoms [19, 26].

Patients may have prodromal fever and malaise, which is more often seen with EM major and occurs less frequently in EM minor, followed by the development of erythematous, edematous papules that favor acral sites although involvement may be generalized [18, 20, 21]. Although EM is classically defined by the presence of target lesions, cutaneous lesions may be varied and include erythematous macules, papules, vesicles, and bullae, differing between patients and evolving throughout the course of presentation [18]. Lesions rapidly progress, and many, although not all, will reach the classic target morphology characterized by three concentric zones of color change: a dusky center surrounded by a pale, edematous ring, and finally an annular, erythematous rim at the periphery [18, 21]. Lesions may coalesce producing a polycyclic or annular appearance [18]. Atypical target lesions may also been seen, defined by only two different colors and a less well-defined border [19, 21]. Lesions may be painful, and less commonly pruritic. While any mucosal site may be involved, oral mucosa is most common and may occur in conjunction with, before, or after the cutaneous eruption. Mucosal lesions are present in 25–60 % of cases, beginning as erythematous vesicles or bullae that quickly progress to painful erosions with hemorrhagic crust, with involvement of two or more mucosal surfaces defining EM major [18, 21]. Ophthalmologic involvement has been reported more frequently in association with infection-related EM than drug-induced EM [27].

Recurrent EM is common, reported in 22–37 % of cases, and most commonly associated with HSV [18, 22, 28]. Mycoplasma-associated EM may present with more severe mucosal involvement and bullous cutaneous eruptions [22]. Some authors suggest the term "*Mycoplasma*-induced rash and mucositis (MIRM)" to describe this subset of patients who typically have significant mucositis and minimal cutaneous involvement [29]. Persistent EM is a rare subtype defined by continuous mucosal and/or cutaneous EM lesions, which is most often associated with underlying viral infection [21].

Laboratory tests are directed by history and examination findings. If there is concern for HSV, viral studies for HSV types 1 and 2 should be performed [21]. Mycoplasma serology and PCR of throat swab may be considered, especially in cases of severe mucositis, along with cold agglutinins and chest X-ray. In severe cases patients may have elevated ESR, lymphocytosis, and transaminitis [21]. Persistent EM has been associated with low complement levels, and, although rare, if EM is persistent or recurrent without an identifiable trigger, evaluation for underlying malignancy should be performed [21].

EM is diagnosed clinically and biopsy is not generally necessary. Histopathology is characterized by interface dermatitis with basal vacuolar degeneration, dyskeratosis, and superficial perivascular lymphocytic infiltrate. Subepidermal bullae may form secondary to vacuolization of the basal layer [21]. Direct immunofluorescence (DIF) may be performed to rule out other diagnoses, as it is usually nonspecific in EM [21]. Of note, histopathology does not reliably distinguish EM from SJS/TEN; thus differentiation between these conditions must be made on clinical grounds.

The differential diagnosis should include SJS/TEN, which may initially appear with atypical targetoid lesions and erythematous macules with dusky centers, as well as conjunctival and mucosal involvement. SJS/TEN is further distinguished by the development of large bullae that easily slough, leaving widespread areas of full-thickness skin denudation. When there is extensive mucosal involvement or bullae formation the differential may include auto-immune bullous disease (e.g., pemphigus, pemphigoid), which can be diagnosed with indirect immunofluorescence (IIF) studies or skin biopsy for DIF [21]. Viral exanthems such as hand-foot-and-mouth disease or primary varicella infection should also be considered, especially if patients complain of a non-specific prodrome of fever and malaise. Urticaria and urticaria multiforme may be confused with early EM, however these lesions are evanescent and fail to exhibit true targets. Vasculitis, Sweet's syndrome, serum-sickness like reaction, and Kawasaki disease are also considered in a child with fever, malaise, arthralgias, and erythematous papular eruption involving the acral surfaces. Systemic lupus erythematous may present with EM-like lesions, which characterizes Rowell's syndrome, for which an anti-nuclear antibody (ANA) titer should be obtained. Fixed-drug eruption may occasionally present with multiple lesions; however there are no true target lesions (Fig. 5.4).

Fig. 5.4 Fixed drug
eruption showing a
well-defined round dusky
patch with two zones of
color change

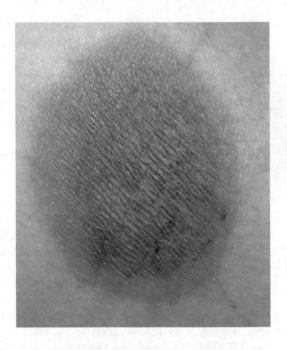

Treatment

EM is self-limited with lesions resolving over 2–4 weeks [18, 20]. Treatment
includes supportive care, appropriate antimicrobials if infection is identified (e.g.,
HSV, mycoplasma), and withdrawal of any potentially inciting medication. EM
minor generally runs a mild course, and treatment is directed toward symptomatic
care with topical corticosteroids and oral antihistamines for pruritus.

EM major may require more aggressive local wound care as well as pain-control
for severe mucositis. Oral swish-and-spit preparations containing viscous lidocaine,
antacid, and diphenhydramine may provide relief. If there is ocular involvement,
Ophthalmology should be consulted early in the patient's course given potential for
scarring and long-term sequelae [21, 24, 27]. Mucositis in EM major may lead to
scarring of mucosal surfaces with potential stricture formation of the oral cavity,
trachea, esophagus, and urethra. Physical exam and symptoms should guide further
consultation with ENT or Urology. Although controversial, systemic corticosteroids are sometimes considered for the treatment of severe EM, especially in the
setting of painful mucositis [21]. Randomized controlled trials are lacking, and in
general the risks and benefits of oral corticosteroid use must be carefully weighed
in the setting of potential infection [30]. If employed, systemic steroids are likely
best given early in the course of illness.

If patients have frequent recurrences, anti-viral prophylaxis may be recommended. Refractory cases have been treated with azathioprine, mycophenolate
mofetil, dapsone, immunoglobulin, hydroxychloroquine, thalidomide, and cyclosporine [21].

Case 5.4

History

A 16-year-old female was admitted for a rash that started 4 days prior to admission. The patient endorsed a history of dysuria and low-grade fever 2 weeks ago, for which she was prescribed a 7-day course of trimethoprim-sulfamethoxazole for urinary tract infection by an outside urgent care. Three days after finishing her course of antibiotic, she developed a rash on her face and chest. She presented to an outside hospital and was transferred for further care. Over the next few days the rash progressed to the rest of her body, and she developed erosions of the lips along with high fever, sore throat, and inability to tolerate PO. In addition to those medications mentioned above she endorsed taking acetaminophen and phenazopyridine for her urinary symptoms. This was her first exposure to trimethoprim-sulfamethoxazole.

Physical Examination (Fig. 5.5)

Laboratory

- CBC unremarkable except for Hgb 10.6 g/dL (L) and Hct 31.9% (L)
- Na 141 mEq/L
- K 4.1 mEq/L
- Chloride 113 mEq/L (H)
- CO_2 total 15 mEq/L (L)
- BUN 20 mg/dL
- Cr 2.38 mg/dL (H)
- AST 96 μ/L (H)
- ALT 46 μ/L (H)
- Glucose 136 mg/dL (H)

Biopsy

- Fresh frozen section, roof of blister: full thickness epidermal necrosis
- Permanent section: subepidermal blister with full thickness necrosis, minimal inflammatory infiltrate

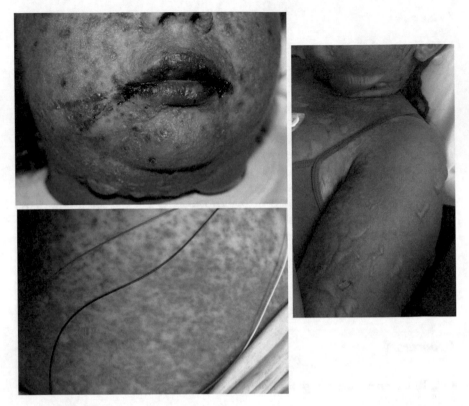

Fig. 5.5 Vital signs were significant for fever to 102.6 F, HR 138, and BP 108/62. She was ill appearing and in obvious pain. Skin examination showed large confluent dusky and violaceous patches and flaccid bullae with areas of full-thickness skin detachment involving her face, neck, chest, abdomen, back, arms, and legs. Estimated body surface area involved was 75%. Nikolsky sign was positive. Conjunctivae were injected, and vermillion lips had hemorrhagic crusting. Genital examination revealed erosions of the labia as well as the perianal skin

Questions

1. What is the differential diagnosis for this eruption?
2. What features in the history, physical, and laboratory/pathology help to make the diagnosis?
3. How might you manage this condition?

Answer

Stevens–Johnson Syndrome (SJS) and Toxic Epidermal Necrolysis (TEN) are severe, life-threatening mucocutaneous hypersensitivity reactions representing a continuum that is graded by extent of cutaneous involvement. Incidence in children is estimated at 0.5 cases per million person-years [31]. Mortality is estimated at 1–5% for SJS and 25–35% for TEN in adults; however, lower rates have been described in children [24, 32–35].

SJS/TEN is primarily caused by drugs; however, reports also document mycoplasma pneumonia and HSV as inciting triggers. Mycoplasma is reported to be a major cause of SJS in children, while medications remain the primary trigger for TEN in children and adults alike [2, 24, 34, 35]. The most common culprit drugs are antimicrobials, specifically sulfonamides (as in this case), aromatic anticonvulsants, benzodiazepines, NSAIDS, corticosteroids, and chemotherapeutic agents [8, 32, 36].

SJS/TEN represents an immunologic reaction to a triggering antigen. Cytotoxic T-cell activation and subsequent release of cell-death mediators including granzyme B, perforin, tumor necrosis factor-alpha (TNF-α), as well as increased Fas-Fas ligand interaction, culminate in keratinocyte apoptosis and epidermal necrosis [31, 37, 38]. There is evidence to support genetic linkages between HLA type and specific drugs in the development of SJS/TEN. For example, HLA-B1502 has been associated with the development of SJS/TEN after exposure to carbamazepine in the Han Chinese population [32, 37, 39]. Recurrent SJS was found in one in five children in a study conducted by two large pediatric tertiary referral centers, which the study concluded may be suggestive of a genetic predisposition in certain individuals [40].

Clinical manifestations of SJS/TEN usually begin within 1–3 weeks of medication exposure. Symptoms may be insidious at onset, with fever, eye discomfort, and dysphagia, followed by the development of erythematous-to-dusky macules on the face and trunk, painful erythroderma, and hemorrhagic erosions of the mucosal surfaces. The development of bullae and epidermal sloughing with slight lateral pressure defines the Nikolsky sign. The extent of cutaneous involvement determines diagnosis: <10% body surface area (BSA) in SJS, >10% and <30% BSA in SJS/TEN overlap, and >30% BSA in TEN [2, 32, 35, 38]. Patients initially presenting with SJS may rapidly evolve to TEN. Ocular involvement generally manifests as severe, exudative conjunctivitis. Mucosal erosions may affect the lips, tongue, buccal mucosa, eyes, nose, genitalia, and rectum. Less commonly mucosal sloughing extends to the esophageal or respiratory epithelium, thus necessitating mechanical ventilation [2, 31]. Some patients may develop even more profound systemic symptoms leading to renal failure, hepatitis, myocarditis, pneumonitis, arthritis, and/or septicemia [2, 31].

The diagnosis is made clinically although skin biopsy is generally recommended to confirm diagnosis. Histopathology of SJS and TEN exists on a continuum, and differentiation between these entities requires clinical correlation. SJS shows a lymphocytic interface dermatitis with necrotic keratinocytes, while specimens from TEN usually reveal full-thickness epidermal necrosis and subepidermal bullae [37]. Two biopsy specimens should be obtained, one for standard formalin fixation and a second for frozen section analysis to allow for more rapid diagnosis [37, 38].

The differential diagnosis of SJS/TEN may include Staphylococcal Scalded Skin Syndrome (SSSS), Kawasaki disease, EM, autoimmune bullous diseases, and

Drug Reaction with Eosinophilia and Systemic Symptoms (DRESS). Children with Kawasaki disease usually have non-purulent conjunctivitis and do not develop bullae or sloughing of mucous membranes. Atypical targetoid cutaneous lesions and mucosal erosions may lead to the consideration of EM; however, the latter is by definition less extensive, is characterized by true target lesions, and is more commonly triggered by infection than medication [2]. TEN is distinguished from autoimmune bullous disease, such as linear IgA bullous dermatosis, bullous pemphigoid, or pemphigus vulgaris, based on negative direct immunofluorescence (DIF) on perilesional skin biopsy, indirect immunofluorescence (IIF) serum studies, and the severe systemic symptoms seen in SJS/TEN that are less commonly associated with immunobullous disease. In SSSS, mucous membranes are spared and the epidermal detachment is superficial compared to the full-thickness skin loss in TEN [2, 31]. The cutaneous morphology of DRESS syndrome may be highly varied although DRESS does not involve mucous membranes and histopathology in DRESS is not characterized by epidermal necrosis [31]. Early SJS/TEN may appear similar to an exanthematous or morbilliform drug eruption; however, the former will involve mucous membranes and rapidly evolve to dusky macules and bullae with epidermal sloughing [39]. TEN-like eruptions have also been observed in patients with systemic lupus erythematosus as well as graft-versus-host disease [39, 41–44].

The most important aspect of management in SJS/TEN is rapid diagnosis and subsequent identification and removal of the offending agent. SCORTEN is a prognostication tool based on age, presence of malignancy, BSA involved, tachycardia, and serum glucose, bicarbonate, and urea values [32]. This predictive tool has been used to assess mortality in adults; however, it has not been validated in a pediatric population [2, 36, 37]. Recently published data found SCORTEN to be predictive of morbidity in pediatric SJS/TEN, with higher scores indicating longer admission, increased time until re-epithelialization, longer duration of mechanical ventilation, greater requirement for surgical procedures, and increased number of infectious complications [45].

Patients should be managed in a burn or pediatric intensive care unit, with early transfer associated with decreased morbidity and mortality [35]. Compromised epidermal barrier in SJS/TEN leads to thermoregulatory instability, electrolyte abnormalities, dehydration, and sepsis. Stringent wound care is of the utmost importance with non-stick, biologic dressings. Systemic antibiotics are indicated if there is clinical or microbiologic evidence of wound infection [2, 31, 38]. Ophthalmology should be consulted expediently for evaluation given potential for ocular sequelae, which occurs in 40–73 % of patients and may result in permanent visual loss [2, 32, 33, 35, 37]. Cutaneous lesions usually heal without scarring although patients may have persistent dyspigmentation or nail dystrophy [2, 35, 39, 46]. Stricture formation may result if there is involvement of esophageal, genital, or anal mucosa, thus clinical signs and symptoms should dictate consultation with Urology or surgical colleagues.

Treatment

In general, there is a paucity of evidence-based data, lack of standardized treatment guidelines, and ongoing controversy over appropriate treatment for SJS/TEN. Multiple systemic therapies have been trialed with limited success in the treatment of SJS/TEN [8]. Given that SJS/TEN is a rare disease, with even lower incidence in children, any available evidence on management is largely derived from the adult population, and it remains unclear if this data can be generalized to pediatric cases [36]. Systemic corticosteroids have historically been the standard of care; however, their use is controversial and generally discouraged given lack of evidence for efficacy and concerns regarding impaired wound healing and increased risk of infection [2, 38, 46]. Due to its immunomodulatory effect in inhibiting Fas-mediated keratinocyte apoptosis, pooled intravenous immunoglobulin (IVIG) is currently the most commonly reported treatment for pediatric SJS/TEN, although studies are conflicting on whether there is true survival benefit with this therapy [2, 31, 35, 38]. There are case reports and small case series citing the beneficial use of cyclosporine A, ulinastatin, plasmapheresis, pentoxifylline, and granulocyte colony-stimulating factor (G-CSF) in the treatment of pediatric SJS/TEN, though reports are limited by small patient population and poor data collection [36–38].

In the adult population, cyclosporine, cyclophosphamide, and plasmapheresis have shown efficacy, but there is very limited evidence regarding their use in pediatric cases [2, 37, 38, 46]. Recently, there has been mounting evidence that biological therapy with TNF-α inhibitors (i.e., infliximab, etanercept) may be beneficial in the treatment of SJS/TEN, the pathomechanism of which is supported by the finding of increased levels of TNF-α in serum and lesional skin of patients with SJS/TEN [38]. Additional studies are necessary to further evaluate the currently conflicting data and determine optimal treatment regimen [39].

Case 5.5

History

An 8-year-old girl with dermatomyositis undergoing treatment with prednisone and rituximab was admitted for cutaneous disseminated herpes zoster and started on IV acyclovir with improvement. However, on day 3 of acyclovir, she developed purulent drainage from some of her lesions. Wound culture confirmed oxacillin-resistant *S. aureus*, and IV clindamycin was added for her soft-tissue infection. Six days later, she developed a pruritic rash for which Dermatology was consulted. This rash began on her abdomen and subsequently spread to the rest of the trunk and extremities.

Physical Examination (Fig. 5.6)

Laboratory

- CBC significant for:
- WBC 9.63 K/μL (N)
- Neutrophil 63 % (N)
- Lymphocyte 22 % (L)
- Eosinophil percentage 7.1 % (H)
- Cr and LFT: WNL

Questions

1. What is the usual time frame for appearance of this rash?
2. What is the differential diagnosis for this eruption?

Answer

Morbilliform exanthems are a delayed-type hypersensitivity representing a common form of cutaneous adverse drug reactions [8, 32, 34]. In a multicenter study evaluating cutaneous adverse drug reactions a morbilliform eruption occurred in 30 % of the study population, most commonly triggered by antimicrobials, followed by NSAIDs, barbiturates, and anticonvulsants [10, 32]. These eruptions generally

Fig. 5.6 Erythematous papules and macules with many areas of confluence on the trunk, arms, and legs

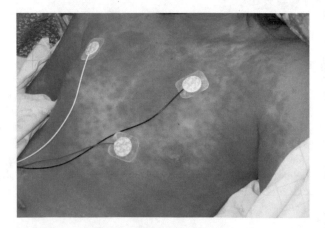

occur 7–14 days after initiation of the culprit drug, and the incidence is increased in patients with concomitant viral infections, specifically Epstein–Barr virus (EBV) infections [8, 34].

The eruption consists of erythematous macules and papules which often, but not always, begin on the trunk and progress to involve the face and extremities. The morbilliform eruption is also commonly referred to as "maculopapular" or "exanthematous." Lesions may coalesce to produce generalized erythroderma, and mucosal surfaces are usually uninvolved. Pruritus is a common complaint. The eruption resolves in approximately 2 weeks with hyperpigmentation and desquamation [8].

A morbilliform morphology can be seen in a variety of other settings, including viral exanthems, Kawasaki disease, toxic shock syndrome, and graft-versus-host disease. Thus, a thorough history and physical examination arc of utmost importance in the evaluation of a morbilliform eruption. At times, the differential diagnosis may also include erythema multiforme, SJS/TEN, and scarlet fever. When a morbilliform eruption is attributed to a drug, the possibility of DRESS syndrome should be ruled out. The latter is a potentially life-threatening drug eruption that presents with fever, facial edema, lymphadenopathy, eosinophilia, and systemic organ involvement with resultant transaminitis, renal dysfunction, and cardiac and thyroid toxicity [7]. Unlike an uncomplicated morbilliform eruption, the development of DRESS syndrome is delayed, with onset generally 2–6 weeks after exposure to the culprit agent [7].

Physical examination and history of recent drug administration can confirm the clinical diagnosis, thus skin biopsy is not routinely needed. Histopathology of morbilliform drug eruption is nonspecific, demonstrating a perivascular lymphocytic infiltrate that may contain eosinophils and scattered necrotic keratinocytes [8]. Therefore, differentiation from a viral exanthem is often impossible on the basis of histopathology alone.

Treatment

Management involves supportive care and discussion of risks and benefits associated with discontinuation of the culprit medication. If possible, discontinuation of the agent with substitution for an alternative is preferred. However, if no reasonable substitution can be made, the drug may be continued with careful monitoring. Oral antihistamines and topical corticosteroids may be employed for symptomatic relief of pruritus [8].

Case 5.6

History

A 6-year-old female was treated with trimethoprim-sulfamethoxazole for a staphylococcus aureus skin infection. Four weeks later she developed a pruritic eruption starting on the arms and generalizing to the rest of her body. She was admitted to an outside hospital and treated with a 3-day course of prednisone. She improved and was discharged home. One day later, she presented to the hospital with a worsening rash, fever, intense pruritus, and complains of abdominal and chest pain. Her parents note her face is swollen and that she has swollen lymph nodes.

Physical Exam (Fig. 5.7)

Laboratory Parameters

- White blood count: 18.7 (4.0–10.5 K/μL)
- Eosinophils 25 % (0–7 %)
- ALT 194 (30–65 U/L)
- AST 87 (15–37 U/L)
- Gamma GT 426 (5–55 U/L)
- Creatinine 0.79 (0.1–1.1 mg/dL)
- Pro-Brain Natriuretic Peptide 2583 (<1318 pg/mL)
- Troponin <0.02 (<0.05 ng/mL)
- Infectious work-up including mycoplasma and hepatitis screen negative
- Chest X-ray, EKG, and echocardiogram negative

Questions

1. What is the differential diagnosis?
2. What treatment would you consider?

Answer

DRESS syndrome (Drug Reaction with Eosinophilia and Systemic Symptoms), also called Drug-Induced Hypersensitivity Syndrome (DIHS), typically presents with an erythematous morbilliform rash that may include the entire skin surface.

Fig. 5.7 Erythematous macules and papules coalescing into ill-defined patches and plaques in a generalized distribution. Her face, hands, and feet are edematous. She has cervical and inguinal lymphadenopathy. Her mucous membranes are intact

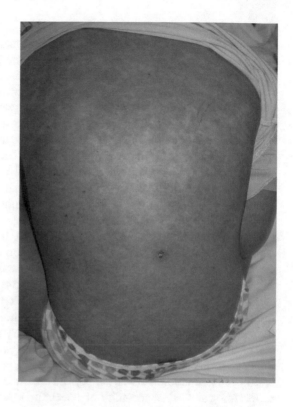

Onset of symptoms is generally 2–6 weeks after drug administration. Facial edema is often noted, with the eruption spreading caudally. The liver is the most commonly affected visceral organ. Inflammation of the heart, lungs, kidney, and central nervous system has been described. Affected patients often demonstrate eosinophilia and atypical lymphocytosis.

There are numerous drugs reported to cause DRESS including aromatic anticonvulsants (carbamazepine, phenytoin, and phenobarbital), sulfonamides, minocycline, lamotrigine, and allopurinol. The diagnosis of DRESS is made from a combination of clinical and laboratory findings. Diagnostic criteria have been proposed by Bocquet et al., the European Registry of Severe Cutaneous Adverse Reaction study group, and the Japanese Research Committee on Severe Cutaneous Adverse Reaction group, and all include the presence of an acute rash, fever, lymphadenopathy, internal organ involvement, and hematologic abnormalities [47–49]. The mortality rate is thought to be 5–10 % [50].

The differential diagnosis includes other drug eruptions such as simple drug hypersensitivity without organ involvement, viral exanthems such as HHV-6, EBV, CMV, Hepatitis A, Hepatitis B, influenza, primary HIV, hypereosinophilic syndrome, Kikuchi syndrome, and lymphoma. Other diseases with rash, multiorgan involvement and eosinophilia are Churg–Strauss, systemic-onset juvenile idiopathic arthritis, and Kawasaki disease. The lack of mucosal involvement of DRESS helps distinguish it from SJS/TEN. DRESS less commonly presents with various cutaneous morphologies, including purpura, chelitis, vesicles, bullae, and targets.

The pathogenesis of DRESS is incompletely understood, with suspected culprits including toxic drug metabolites, viral reactivation, and the subsequent host immune response. Drug detoxification enzyme abnormalities may result in accumulation of toxic drug metabolites. Reactivation of herpes viruses CMV, EBV, VZV, human herpesvirus-6 (HHV-6) and -7 (HHV-7) have been implicated in the pathogenesis, with multiple studies showing serologic evidence that HHV-6 is the first virus reactivated in DRESS [51]. Reports hypothesize that drug metabolites may cause a transient immune suppression which triggers viral reactivation within T-cells. This induces production of antiviral T-cells that produce pro-inflammatory cytokines, resulting in end-organ damage that is most prominent at sites, where the virus has replicated (liver, skin, heart, kidneys) [52, 53]. Activated T-cells also stimulate the development of eosinophils through release of interleukin-5 (IL-5), which may cause further end-organ damage. Yet another component is the identification of genetic predisposition with certain HLA types predisposing individuals to DRESS and other drug hypersensitivity syndromes [51, 54].

Diagnosis is made clinically, and thus skin biopsy is often not necessary unless the cutaneous presentation is atypical. Histopathology is often nonspecific with a perivascular lymphocytic infiltrate in the papillary dermis and variable presence of eosinophils [8]. Laboratory evaluation of patients with DRESS syndrome should include complete blood count with differential, serum chemistry to include renal and hepatic function, as well as thyroid function testing and baseline EKG and echocardiogram [8]. Myocarditis can occur up to 4 months after the acute presentation of DRESS [55]. Thyroid function should be repeated every 2–3 months for at least 1 year, with prolonged assessment for signs or symptoms of thyroid dysfunction as there are reports of late thyroid sequelae occurring between 2 months to 3 years after initial diagnosis of DRESS [56].

Treatment

Treatment involves withdrawal of causative drug and supportive care with topical corticosteroids and antihistamines to help itching in mild cases. In more severe cases with internal organ involvement systemic corticosteroids 1–2 mg/kg/day for 3–4 weeks with gradual taper to prevent rebound is recommended [54]. Most patients have complete recovery after withdrawal of the causative drug. Sequelae from the eruption include an exfoliative dermatitis, and children may have residual skin pigmentary changes. There are reports of treatment with IVIG, plasmapheresis, systemic immunosuppressives, and anti-herpesvirus medications [57]. Further studies are required on the effectiveness of treatments.

Case 5.7

History

A 9-year-old female with past medical history significant for seizure disorder was admitted for fever and rash. Five days prior to admission she presented to her pediatrician with sore throat and was prescribed amoxicillin. On day 4 of antibiotic therapy, she developed a rash that began in her groin area and subsequently spread to her thighs, axillae, and trunk. It was mildly pruritic and she had intermittent low-grade temperatures. She has been on valproic acid for years and has had no recent changes in her seizure medications. The parents denied any recent use of OTC medications at home.

Physical Examination (Fig. 5.8)

Laboratory

- WBC 17.6 (H)
- Hgb 10.3 (L)
- Hct 29.8 (L)
- PTL 268
- Absolute neutrophils 10.5×10^9/L (H)
- Absolute eosinophils: WNL
- LFTs: WNL

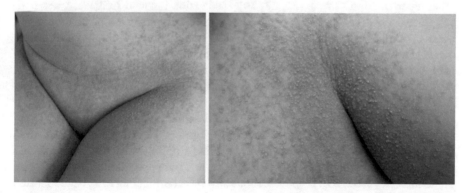

Fig. 5.8 Numerous <1 mm monomorphous superficial pustules with underlying erythema involving the intertriginous areas, including the neck, axillae, and groin. Her mucous membranes were intact

Skin Biopsy

- Spongiosis in the epidermis and subcorneal collections of neutrophils forming a pustule.

Questions

1. What are the most common causes of this eruption, and what is the usual time frame for appearance of rash?
2. What is the differential diagnosis for this widespread pustular eruption?

Answer

Acute generalized exanthematous pustulosis (AGEP) is a pustular hypersensitivity reaction that is uncommon in the pediatric population [32]. Though pathogenesis is unclear AGEP is thought to be a delayed-type hypersensitivity reaction to drug exposure involving T-cell-mediated keratinocyte destruction and/or deposition of drug or infection-induced antigen-antibody complexes [19, 32, 58, 59]. Unlike the adult population, in which medications are the primary culprit, AGEP in children may be secondary to viral (e.g., adenovirus, enterovirus, parvovirus, Coxsackie virus, CMV, EBV, hepatitis B virus) as well as bacterial infections (e.g., *Mycoplasma pneumoniae*) [2, 8, 32, 58, 59]. Commonly implicated medications include Beta-lactam antibiotics, macrolides, clindamycin, and vancomycin, among numerous other reported culprit drugs [32, 58, 59]. Medication-induced AGEP characteristically occurs within the first 1–5 days of therapy, at times even occurring within hours of medication exposure. Its rapid onset in the course of drug administration can aid in distinguishing from other drug eruptions [8, 58, 60]. There are reports related to vaccine administration, mercury exposure, and IV contrast [58, 60, 61]. Although at times severe in its clinical presentation, mortality in AGEP remains less than 5 % [32].

AGEP presents with the acute development of hundreds of diffusely scattered, sterile, non-follicular-based pustules on a background of intense erythema, often most notable in intertriginous areas [8, 59]. The eruption is usually accompanied by fever, and laboratory evaluation often shows lymphocytosis with neutrophil predominance [8, 32, 59]. Hypocalcemia and hypoalbuminemia have been reported [58]. The primary differential diagnosis is acute pustular psoriasis, von Zumbusch type. As compared with pustular psoriasis, AGEP is characterized by more rapid onset, a history of medication exposure or prodromal illness, and at times the presence of variable cutaneous morphologies including purpura, vesicles, bullae, or target lesions, which are not characteristic of pustular psoriasis [7, 19, 58].

The differential also includes subcorneal pustular dermatosis although the latter is very rare in the pediatric population. In extensive cases pustules may coalesce leading to the consideration of TEN, although AGEP is not generally associated with mucous membrane involvement and the histopathology of AGEP is distinct from TEN. DRESS syndrome with pustules is also considered; however, unlike AGEP, DRESS occurs at a prolonged interval after medication exposure and is characterized by facial edema, lymphadenopathy, eosinophilia, and transaminitis [19]. Pustular miliaria may be confused with early AGEP although miliaria lacks progression or systemic symptoms, and there is often history of excessive heat or occlusion of the involved area.

A CBC, complete metabolic panel, and skin biopsy are recommended in the evaluation of AGEP. Bacterial culture may be considered if other infectious etiology is suspected and will be sterile in AGEP [60]. Histopathology of AGEP shows intra-epidermal or subcorneal pustules, papillary dermal edema, and perivascular infiltrates containing eosinophils and neutrophils [2, 7, 32]. Leukocytoclastic vasculitis and focal keratinocyte necrosis are less commonly seen [19, 58]. On biopsy pustular psoriasis may demonstrate identical pustule formation to that seen in AGEP; however, the former may also demonstrate features consistent with classic psoriasis such as papillomatosis and epidermal acanthosis, which assists in differentiation [58].

Treatment

Primary treatment is removal of the offending agent in medication-induced eruptions and supportive care. Pustules resolve in 1–2 weeks with resultant superficial desquamation [8, 59]. Topical corticosteroids and antihistamines may aid in relief of pruritus if present, and a short course of oral corticosteroids may hasten resolution in severe cases [8, 32].

Case 5.8

History

A 17-year-old female with well-controlled type I diabetes was admitted for workup of painful skin lesions. These first appeared 3 weeks prior on the shins but subsequently worsened and spread to her feet, thighs, and to a lesser extent her arms. They are very painful, and over the past 3 days she has been unable to ambulate due to pain. There has been no change in her insulin regimen for the past year. Her only new medication is an oral contraceptive pill, which was started 3 months ago. She reports no recent fever, malaise, sore throat, cough, rhinorrhea, chest pain, abdominal pain, vomiting, diarrhea, dysuria, or joint pains.

Physical Examination (Fig. 5.9)

Laboratory

- CBC and CMP were unremarkable
- ESR 35 mm/h (H)
- ASO 200 IU (N)
- Rapid strep negative
- Urinalysis unremarkable
- CXR unremarkable

Skin Biopsy

- Septal panniculitis with superficial and deep lymphocytic inflammation.

Questions

1. What is the differential diagnosis of EN?
2. What are potential triggers of EN?

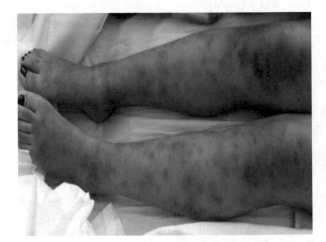

Fig. 5.9 Numerous erythematous, ill-defined, exquisitely tender, deep-seated nodules on the feet, legs, thighs, and to a lesser extent the arms. Photo courtesy of Ashley Crew, MD

Answer

Erythema nodosum (EN) is a cutaneous hypersensitivity reaction characterized by erythematous, tender, subcutaneous nodules and represents the most common form of panniculitis in children [2, 60, 62, 63]. EN is most often seen in adolescents and rarely reported in those under 2 years of age. There is slight female predominance in postpubertal cases with equal sex distribution in prepubertal patients [60, 64]. Lesions classically occur symmetrically on the pretibial surfaces in adults, but in children may be more generalized, extending to thighs, arms, and face [2, 62, 65]. Tender, erythematous, ovoid nodules, 1–6 cm in diameter with poorly defined borders are characteristic, which resolve over days to weeks with hyperpigmentation or ecchymotic-appearing patches without scarring [2, 63]. New lesions may continue to develop with the entire eruption resolving over 3–6 weeks, with reports citing shorter duration in children [64, 66]. The onset of cutaneous lesions is often associated with fever and malaise. Arthralgias are a common feature in adults, but less commonly reported in children [2, 60, 63, 65]. A variant of EN involving the palms and soles has been reported in children, which presents after physical activity as unilateral, erythematous nodules, biopsies of which are consistent with EN [63].

The pathogenesis of EN is related to an immune-mediated delayed hypersensitivity reaction to a variety of antigens, causing immune complex deposition in small vessels of the reticular dermis and subcutaneous fat [63]. This activates the complement cascade, releasing pro-inflammatory mediators and resulting in local edema, erythema, and pain [60]. In greater than 50 % of cases EN is idiopathic, although the most common identifiable trigger in pediatric cases is streptococcal pharyngitis [2, 60, 64, 65]. There are reports of associations with multiple infectious agents, most commonly *Mycoplasma pneumoniae*, *Yersinia enterocolitica*, *Chlamydia pneumoniae*, respiratory viruses, Epstein–Barr virus (EBV), mycobacteria, coccidiomycosis, and giardia. Potential culprit drugs include oral contraceptives, cephalosporins, penicillin, macrolides, sulfonamides, NSAIDs, bromides, and iodides, to name just a few among the lengthy list of implicated drugs [63, 67]. EN has also been associated with inflammatory diseases, in particular inflammatory bowel disease, sarcoidosis, Behcet's disease, and collagen vascular disease, as well as pregnancy and malignancy [2, 64].

The clinical presentation is often quite characteristic although the differential diagnosis includes cellulitis or erysipelas, deep fungal infections, arthropod assault, cutaneous vasculitis, and other panniculitis [2, 68]. Cellulitis is usually localized to one site and is uncommonly bilateral although it may be similarly associated with fever, systemic symptoms, and lymphocytosis. Deep fungal infection would be considered in an immunocompromised patient and may necessitate biopsy for tissue culture. Arthropod assault may be determined by close inspection for central punctum and linear groupings as well as primary complaint of pruritus, which contrasts with the prominent pain seen in EN. Leukocytoclastic vasculitis presents with palpable purpura on the lower legs with proximal progression. Cutaneous polyarteritis nodosa also manifests as tender, erythematous subcutaneous nodules, often associated with livedo reticularis and systemic symptoms. Histopathology differentiates this entity from EN by demonstration of a neutrophilic, necrotizing vasculitis of small- and medium-sized arteries [67, 69]. Other cutaneous vasculitides, such as Henoch–Schönlein purpura, often present with palpable purpura, however can be difficult to differentiate clinically from EN and may warrant biopsy [60, 65, 70]. Erythema induratum (nodular vasculitis) more commonly presents on the posterior calves with ulceration and subsequent scarring, with biopsy showing lobular or mixed panniculitis with vasculitis [2, 19, 68]. Cold-induced panniculitis presents on cheeks and outer thighs, while lupus panniculitis often involves upper arms and face, with biopsy showing lobular panniculitis, which allows further discernment from EN [60, 67, 70].

Patients may have leukocytosis and elevated ESR. Laboratory evaluation should include CBC, ESR and/or CRP, complete metabolic panel, throat culture, antistreptolysin-O or DNase B titer, urinalysis, chest radiograph, and evaluation for occult tuberculosis infection [62, 63, 68]. Further infectious work-up should be guided by history and associated symptoms and may include serum analyses for Yersinia, chlamydia, mycoplasma, viral infections, and/or stool ova and parasite examination [2, 60, 62, 68]. Skin biopsy is not required but may be obtained if the diagnosis is in question or presentation is atypical. On histopathology, EN is prototypically characterized by septal panniculitis with early findings of septal thickening and neutrophilic infiltration, which evolves to a lymphohistiocytic infiltrate with giant cells in established lesions. There is notable absence of vasculitis [19, 63, 68].

Treatment

Treatment is dependent upon the underlying cause, with the treatment of coexisting streptococcal or other infection, if identified, or discontinuation of any potential offending medication. Supportive care is the mainstay of therapy with bed rest for 2–3 days, elevation of the lower extremities, compression, and restriction of physical activity for several weeks, which may prevent recurrence or exacerbation [63, 65]. NSAIDs may be given for pain or arthralgias. Other treatments include colchicine, potassium iodide, or short-course systemic corticosteroids; however, the use of steroids must be carefully considered in the setting of potential infection [2, 60, 68]. Recurrence is possible, and reported as more common in those patients in whom an underlying etiology was not identified, or in which EN was associated with an upper-respiratory tract infection [63, 64].

References

1. Langley EW, Gigante J. Anaphylaxis, urticaria, and angioedema. Pediatr Rev. 2013;34(6):247–57.
2. Paller A, Mancini AJ, Hurwitz S. Hurwitz clinical pediatric dermatology. Edinburgh: Elsevier; 2011. https://libproxy.usc.edu/login?url=http://ZB5LH7ED7A.search.serialssolutions.com/? V=1.0&L=ZB5LH7ED7A&S=JCs&C=TC0000551457&T=marc.
3. Pite H, Wedi B, Borrego LM, Kapp A, Raap U. Management of childhood urticaria: current knowledge and practical recommendations. Acta Derm Venereol. 2013;93(5):500–8.
4. Godse KV, Zawar V, Krupashankar D, Girdhar M, Kandhari S, Dhar S, et al. Consensus statement on the management of urticaria. Indian J Dermatol. 2011;56(5):485–9.
5. Greaves MW. Pathology and classification of urticaria. Immunol Allergy Clin North Am. 2014;34(1):1–9.
6. Mortureux P, Léauté-Labrèze C, Legrain-Lifermann V, Lamireau T, Sarlangue J, Taïeb A. Acute urticaria in infancy and early childhood: a prospective study. Arch Dermatol. 1998;134(3):319–23.
7. Eichenfield LF, Frieden IJ, Mathes EF, Zaenglein AL. Neonatal and infant dermatology. London: Elsevier; 2015. https://libproxy.usc.edu/login?url=http://ZB5LH7ED7A.search.serialssolutions.com/?V=1.0&L=ZB5LH7ED7A&S=JCs&C=TC0001398876&T=marc.
8. Heelan K, Shear NH. Cutaneous drug reactions in children: an update. Paediatr Drugs. 2013;15(6):493–503.
9. Marrouche N, Grattan C. Childhood urticaria. Curr Opin Allergy Clin Immunol. 2012;12(5):485–90.
10. Dilek N, Özkol HU, Akbaş A, Kılınç F, Dilek AR, Saral Y, et al. Cutaneous drug reactions in children: a multicentric study. Postepy Dermatol Alergol. 2014;31(6):368–71.
11. Rosenblatt AE, Stein SL. Cutaneous reactions to vaccinations. Clin Dermatol. 2015;33(3):327–32.
12. Mathur AN, Mathes EF. Urticaria mimickers in children. Dermatol Ther. 2013;26(6):467–75.
13. Sackesen C, Sekerel BE, Orhan F, Kocabas CN, Tuncer A, Adalioglu G. The etiology of different forms of urticaria in childhood. Pediatr Dermatol. 2004;21(2):102–8.
14. Kolivras A, Theunis A, Ferster A, Lipsker D, Sass U, Dussart A, et al. Cryopyrin-associated periodic syndrome: an autoinflammatory disease manifested as neutrophilic urticarial dermatosis with additional perieccrine involvement. J Cutan Pathol. 2011;38(2):202–8.
15. Sarkar S, De A. Urticaria multiforme. Indian Pediatr. 2015;52(7):633.
16. Shah KN, Honig PJ, Yan AC. "Urticaria multiforme": a case series and review of acute annular urticarial hypersensitivity syndromes in children. Pediatrics. 2007;119(5):e1177–83.
17. Emer JJ, Bernardo SG, Kovalerchik O, Ahmad M. Urticaria multiforme. J Clin Aesthet Dermatol. 2013;6(3):34–9.
18. Huff JC, Weston WL, Tonnesen MG. Erythema multiforme: a critical review of characteristics, diagnostic criteria, and causes. J Am Acad Dermatol. 1983;8(6):763–75.
19. Bolognia J, Jorizzo JL, Schaffer JV. Dermatology. Philadelphia: Elsevier; 2012. https://libproxy.usc.edu/login?url=http://ZB5LH7ED7A.search.serialssolutions.com/?V=1.0&L=ZB5LH7ED7A&S=JCs&C=TC0000702199&T=marc.
20. Zaoutis LB, Chiang VW. Comprehensive pediatric hospital medicine. Philadelphia: Mosby/Elsevier; 2007. https://libproxy.usc.edu/login?url=http://ZB5LH7ED7A.search.serialssolutions.com/?V=1.0&L=ZB5LH7ED7A&S=JCs&C=TC0000387293&T=marc.
21. Sokumbi O, Wetter DA. Clinical features, diagnosis, and treatment of erythema multiforme: a review for the practicing dermatologist. Int J Dermatol. 2012;51(8):889–902.
22. Schalock PC, Dinulos JG, Pace N, Schwarzenberger K, Wenger JK. Erythema multiforme due to Mycoplasma pneumoniae infection in two children. Pediatr Dermatol. 2006;23(6):546–55.
23. Keller N, Gilad O, Marom D, Marcus N, Garty BZ. Nonbullous erythema multiforme in hospitalized children: a 10-year survey. Pediatr Dermatol. 2015;32(5):701–3.
24. Forman R, Koren G, Shear NH. Erythema multiforme, Stevens-Johnson syndrome and toxic epidermal necrolysis in children: a review of 10 years' experience. Drug Saf. 2002;25(13):965–72.
25. Katoulis AC, Liakou A, Bozi E, Theodorakis M, Alevizou A, Zafeiraki A, et al. Erythema multiforme following vaccination for human papillomavirus. Dermatology. 2010;220(1):60–2.

26. Auquier-Dunant A, Mockenhaupt M, Naldi L, Correia O, Schröder W, Roujeau JC, et al. Correlations between clinical patterns and causes of erythema multiforme majus, Stevens-Johnson syndrome, and toxic epidermal necrolysis: results of an international prospective study. Arch Dermatol. 2002;138(8):1019–24.
27. Moreau JF, Watson RS, Hartman ME, Linde-Zwirble WT, Ferris LK. Epidemiology of ophthalmologic disease associated with erythema multiforme, Stevens-Johnson syndrome, and toxic epidermal necrolysis in hospitalized children in the United States. Pediatr Dermatol. 2014;31(2):163–8.
28. Weston WL, Morelli JG. Herpes simplex virus-associated erythema multiforme in prepubertal children. Arch Pediatr Adolesc Med. 1997;151(10):1014–6.
29. Canavan TN, Mathes EF, Frieden I, Shinkai K. Mycoplasma pneumoniae-induced rash and mucositis as a syndrome distinct from Stevens-Johnson syndrome and erythema multiforme: a systematic review. J Am Acad Dermatol. 2014;72(2):239–45.
30. Léauté-Labrèze C, Lamireau T, Chawki D, Maleville J, Taïeb A. Diagnosis, classification, and management of erythema multiforme and Stevens-Johnson syndrome. Arch Dis Child. 2000;83(4):347–52.
31. Rizzo JA, Johnson R, Cartie RJ. Pediatric toxic epidermal necrolysis: experience of a tertiary burn center. Pediatr Dermatol. 2015;32(5):704–9.
32. Noguera-Morel L, Hernández-Martín Á, Torrelo A. Cutaneous drug reactions in the pediatric population. Pediatr Clin North Am. 2014;61(2):403–26.
33. Levi N, Bastuji-Garin S, Mockenhaupt M, Roujeau JC, Flahault A, Kelly JP, et al. Medications as risk factors of Stevens-Johnson syndrome and toxic epidermal necrolysis in children: a pooled analysis. Pediatrics. 2009;123(2):e297–304.
34. Khaled A, Kharfi M, Ben Hamida M, El Fekih N, El Aidli S, Zeglaoui F, et al. Cutaneous adverse drug reactions in children. A series of 90 cases. Tunis Med. 2012;90(1):45–50.
35. Quirke KP, Beck A, Gamelli RL, Mosier MJ. A 15-year review of pediatric toxic epidermal necrolysis. J Burn Care Res. 2015;36(1):130–6.
36. Del Pozzo-Magana BR, Lazo-Langner A, Carleton B, Castro-Pastrana LI, Rieder MJ. A systematic review of treatment of drug-induced Stevens-Johnson syndrome and toxic epidermal necrolysis in children. J Popul Ther Clin Pharmacol. 2011;18:e121–33.
37. Koh MJ, Tay YK. An update on Stevens-Johnson syndrome and toxic epidermal necrolysis in children. Curr Opin Pediatr. 2009;21(4):505–10.
38. Worswick S, Cotliar J. Stevens-Johnson syndrome and toxic epidermal necrolysis: a review of treatment options. Dermatol Ther. 2011;24(2):207–18.
39. Schwartz RA, McDonough PH, Lee BW. Toxic epidermal necrolysis: part II. Prognosis, sequelae, diagnosis, differential diagnosis, prevention, and treatment. J Am Acad Dermatol. 2013;69(2):187.e1–16. quiz 203-4.
40. Finkelstein Y, Soon GS, Acuna P, George M, Pope E, Ito S, et al. Recurrence and outcomes of Stevens-Johnson syndrome and toxic epidermal necrolysis in children. Pediatrics. 2011;128(4):723–8.
41. Yildirim Cetin G, Sayar H, Ozkan F, Kurtulus S, Kesici F, Sayarlioglu M. A case of toxic epidermal necrolysis-like skin lesions with systemic lupus erythematosus and review of the literature. Lupus. 2013;22(8):839–46.
42. Villada G, Roujeau JC, Cordonnier C, Bagot M, Kuentz M, Wechsler J, et al. Toxic epidermal necrolysis after bone marrow transplantation: study of nine cases. J Am Acad Dermatol. 1990;23(5 Pt 1):870–5.
43. Macedo FI, Faris J, Lum LG, Gabali A, Uberti JP, Ratanatharathorn V, et al. Extensive toxic epidermal necrolysis versus acute graft versus host disease after allogenic hematopoietic stem-cell transplantation: challenges in diagnosis and management. J Burn Care Res. 2014;35(6):e431–5.
44. Jeanmonod P, Hubbuch M, Grünhage F, Meiser A, Rass K, Schilling MK, et al. Graft-versus-host disease or toxic epidermal necrolysis: diagnostic dilemma after liver transplantation. Transpl Infect Dis. 2012;14(4):422–6.
45. Beck A, Quirke KP, Gamelli RL, Mosier MJ. Pediatric toxic epidermal necrolysis: using SCORTEN and predictive models to predict morbidity when a focus on mortality is not enough. J Burn Care Res. 2015;36(1):167–77.

46. Spies M, Sanford AP, Aili Low JF, Wolf SE, Herndon DN. Treatment of extensive toxic epidermal necrolysis in children. Pediatrics. 2001;108(5):1162–8.
47. Bocquet H, Bagot M, Roujeau JC. Drug-induced pseudolymphoma and drug hypersensitivity syndrome (Drug Rash with Eosinophilia and Systemic Symptoms: DRESS). Semin Cutan Med Surg. 1996;15(4):250–7.
48. Kardaun SH, Sidoroff A, Valeyrie-Allanore L, Halevy S, Davidovici BB, Mockenhaupt M, et al. Variability in the clinical pattern of cutaneous side-effects of drugs with systemic symptoms: does a DRESS syndrome really exist? Br J Dermatol. 2007;156(3):609–11.
49. Shiohara T, Iijima M, Ikezawa Z, Hashimoto K. The diagnosis of a DRESS syndrome has been sufficiently established on the basis of typical clinical features and viral reactivations. Br J Dermatol. 2007;156(5):1083–4.
50. Belver MT, Michavila A, Bobolea I, Feito M, Bellón T, Quirce S. Severe delayed skin reactions related to drugs in the paediatric age group: a review of the subject by way of three cases (Stevens-Johnson syndrome, toxic epidermal necrolysis and DRESS). Allergol Immunopathol (Madr). 2016;44(1):83–95.
51. Camous X, Calbo S, Picard D, Musette P. Drug reaction with eosinophilia and systemic symptoms: an update on pathogenesis. Curr Opin Immunol. 2012;24(6):730–5.
52. Cacoub P, Musette P, Descamps V, Meyer O, Speirs C, Finzi L, et al. The DRESS syndrome: a literature review. Am J Med. 2011;124(7):588–97.
53. Walsh SA, Creamer D. Drug reaction with eosinophilia and systemic symptoms (DRESS): a clinical update and review of current thinking. Clin Exp Dermatol. 2011;36(1):6–11.
54. Husain Z, Reddy BY, Schwartz RA. DRESS syndrome: part I. Clinical perspectives. J Am Acad Dermatol. 2013;68(5):693.e1–14. quiz 706-8.
55. Thankachen J, Agarwal V. Challenges in diagnosis, management, and treatment of allopurinol-induced DRESS syndrome: case report and literature review. Am J Ther. 2015;22(3):e77–83.
56. Kano Y, Tohyama M, Aihara M, Matsukura S, Watanabe H, Sueki H, et al. Sequelae in 145 patients with drug-induced hypersensitivity syndrome/drug reaction with eosinophilia and systemic symptoms: survey conducted by the Asian Research Committee on Severe Cutaneous Adverse Reactions (ASCAR). J Dermatol. 2015;42(3):276–82.
57. Alexander T, Iglesia E, Park Y, Duncan D, Peden D, Sheikh S, et al. Severe DRESS syndrome managed with therapeutic plasma exchange. Pediatrics. 2013;131(3):e945–9.
58. Meadows KP, Egan CA, Vanderhooft S. Acute generalized exanthematous pustulosis (AGEP), an uncommon condition in children: case report and review of the literature. Pediatr Dermatol. 2000;17(5):399–402.
59. Ersoy S, Paller AS, Mancini AJ. Acute generalized exanthematous pustulosis in children. Arch Dermatol. 2004;140(9):1172–3.
60. Shin HT, Chang MW. Drug eruptions in children. Curr Probl Pediatr. 2001;31(7):207–34.
61. Hammerbeck AA, Daniels NH, Callen JP. Ioversol-induced acute generalized exanthematous pustulosis: a case report. Arch Dermatol. 2009;145(6):683–7.
62. Torrelo A, Hernández A. Panniculitis in children. Dermatol Clin. 2008;26(4):491–500. vii.
63. Requena L, Yus ES. Erythema nodosum. Dermatol Clin. 2008;26(4):425–38. v.
64. Aydın-Teke T, Tanır G, Bayhan GI, Metin O, Oz N. Erythema nodosum in children: evaluation of 39 patients. Turk J Pediatr. 2014;56(2):144–9.
65. Kakourou T, Drosatou P, Psychou F, Aroni K, Nicolaidou P. Erythema nodosum in children: a prospective study. J Am Acad Dermatol. 2001;44(1):17–21.
66. Cengiz AB, Kara A, Kanra G, Seçmeer G, Ceyhan M. Erythema nodosum in childhood: evaluation of ten patients. Turk J Pediatr. 2006;48(1):38–42.
67. Polcari IC, Stein SL. Panniculitis in childhood. Dermatol Ther. 2010;23(4):356–67.
68. Blake T, Manahan M, Rodins K. Erythema nodosum—a review of an uncommon panniculitis. Dermatol Online J. 2014;20(4):22376.
69. Fathalla BM, Miller L, Brady S, Schaller JG. Cutaneous polyarteritis nodosa in children. J Am Acad Dermatol. 2005;53(4):724–8.
70. Labbé L, Perel Y, Maleville J, Taïeb A. Erythema nodosum in children: a study of 27 patients. Pediatr Dermatol. 1996;13(6):447–50.

Chapter 6
Acute and Chronic Graft-Versus-Host Disease of the Skin

Hasan Khosravi, Anar Mikailov, and Jennifer T. Huang

Abstract Graft-versus-host disease (GVHD) is one of the most challenging diseases to diagnose and manage in both children and adults. Despite significant research and advances, GVHD remains a significant cause of morbidity and mortality in the post-hematopoietic stem cell transplant population. Given that skin is the most common organ affected in both acute and chronic forms of GVHD, it is imperative for dermatologists not only to recognize cutaneous manifestations but also to familiarize themselves with first-line therapies for these conditions. In this chapter, we describe four unique cases of acute and chronic GVHD, and discuss the differential diagnosis, diagnostic pearls, and therapeutic approach to these diseases. We begin with a case of classic acute GVHD, and review characteristic clinical features, risk factors, differential diagnosis, and first-line therapies. We then move on to a rare case of toxic epidermal necrolysis-like acute GVHD and discuss second- and third-line agents for treatment-refractory disease, including interventions that saved the patient's life. In case 3, we transition to a discussion of chronic GVHD, and present a patient with sclerotic disease, reviewing clinical features, risk factors, and first-line therapies for this condition. Lastly, we conclude our chapter with a discussion of an atypical nonsclerotic form cutaneous chronic GVHD associated with a good prognosis.

Keywords Graft-versus-host disease • Pediatric graft-versus-host disease • Hematopoietic stem cell transplant • Bone marrow transplant • GVHD • Acute GVHD • Chronic GVHD

H. Khosravi, BS
Harvard Medical School, Boston, MA, USA

A. Mikailov, MD
Harvard Combined Medicine-Dermatology Residency Program, Boston, MA, USA

J.T. Huang, MD (✉)
Dermatology Program, Boston Children's Hospital, Harvard Medical School,
300 Longwood Avenue, Boston, MA, USA
e-mail: Jennifer.huang@childrens.harvard.edu

© Springer International Publishing Switzerland 2016
M. Hogeling (ed.), *Case-Based Inpatient Pediatric Dermatology*,
DOI 10.1007/978-3-319-31569-0_6

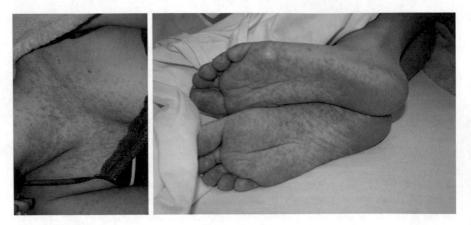

Fig. 6.1 Scattered 1–2 mm erythematous macules and papules scattered on face, trunk, and extremities with involvement of palms and soles consistent with acute GVHD of the skin

Case 6.1. Acute Graft-Versus-Host Disease

Presentation

A 19-year-old girl who underwent a fully matched unrelated donor bone marrow hematopoietic stem cell transplant (HSCT) for acute myeloid leukemia (AML) presented with a full body rash 33 days after HSCT. The new rash was first noted at 31 days after HSCT, initially involving the chest with subsequent spread to the face, arms, and legs. She endorsed mild pruritus, and denied skin tenderness, eye discomfort, or dysuria. She denied any new medications in the last 2 weeks, upper respiratory symptoms, or any sick contacts. She denied abdominal pain, diarrhea, nausea, or vomiting. She had received systemic corticosteroids, cyclosporine, and short course of high dose methotrexate for prophylaxis against graft-versus-host disease (GVHD).

Physical Exam

On physical examination, the patient appeared ill but in no acute distress. There were scattered 1–2 mm erythematous macules and papules predominantly on the central chest, upper back, face, ears, palms, soles, and legs (Fig. 6.1). There was no involvement of the oral or ocular mucosa.

Labs

- Aspartate aminotransferase (AST) 72 unit/L (10–40 IU/L)
- Alanine transaminase (ALT) 196 μ/L (7–56 IU/L)
- Total bilirubin 0.8 mg/dL (0.3–1.2 mg/dL)
- Blood urea nitrogen (BUN) 19 mg/dL (5–18 mg/dL)
- Creatinine 0.8 mg/dL (0.5–1.2 mg/dL)

Questions

1. What are the risk factors for acute cutaneous GVHD in children?
2. What are the classic morphologic patterns of acute GVHD? What are the other primary clinical features?
3. What is the differential diagnosis for acute GVHD and what is the utility of skin biopsy?
4. What is the treatment plan?
5. What is the prognosis for children with acute cutaneous GVHD?

Discussion

Pediatric Acute GVHD Risk Factors

The most important risk factor for acute GVHD in children is human leukocyte antigen (HLA) disparity. Recent data from the National Marrow Donor Program showed an incidence of acute GVHD grade II–IV of 40–85 % among unrelated donor, bone marrow HSCT, compared to an incidence of 28 % in HLA-identical sibling bone marrow HSCT [1]. Advances in high resolution HLA matching (10 alleles) has significantly decreased rates of high-grade acute cutaneous GVHD from 30 to 50 % to about 8 % [1]. Stem cell source is also an important factor in determining a child's risk for acute GVHD. Due to the immunologic naïveté and adaptability of umbilical cord blood, more HLA disparity is permissible with use of cord blood over bone marrow. Thus there is a similar incidence of acute GVHD in those who receive 4/6 HLA-matched cord blood HSCT and those who receive a fully matched bone marrow HSCT [1]. Other well-established high risk factors for acute GVHD in children include older donor age and sex mismatch (multiparous female donor to male recipient is the highest risk) [1, 2].

Clinical Presentation of Acute Cutaneous GVHD

Acute GVHD was originally distinguished from chronic GVHD by classic signs and symptoms that presented within 100 days of HSCT, though recent guidelines from the National Institutes of Health deemphasize time-based criteria and instead place much more importance on clinical findings [3]. Skin is the most commonly affected organ, followed by the gastrointestinal tract and liver [4, 5]. Gastrointestinal involvement is measured by 24 h stool output, and liver involvement by bilirubin levels. Earliest cutaneous findings include erythema or purple discoloration of the ears, face, palms, and soles [5, 6]. This is followed by erythematous macules coalescing into patches with folliculocentric prominence and symmetrical distribution. While pruritus is a common symptom, skin tenderness or pain is not uncommon and can be an ominous sign of progressive disease. The most severe presentation of acute cutaneous GVHD includes erythroderma, bullae and/or sloughing, reminiscent of toxic epidermal necrolysis (TEN). Additionally, like TEN, severe acute cutaneous GVHD can involve the mucosal membranes including the eyes and genitalia—further discussion in Case 6.2. The current case was clinically consistent with mild acute GVHD based on the cutaneous findings (Fig. 1.1) along with elevated hepatic inflammatory markers.

Differential Diagnosis and the Utility of Skin Biopsy

The differential diagnosis for acute cutaneous GVHD includes engraftment syndrome, toxic erythema of chemotherapy, viral exanthem, and drug hypersensitivity [5, 6]. Engraftment syndrome presents within 1–2 weeks after HSCT with fever, morbilliform eruption, and edema. Lung involvement, including pulmonary edema, is characteristic. This presentation rapidly responds to systemic corticosteroids. Toxic erythema of chemotherapy can present during conditioning and up to 3 weeks after transplant. Findings are variable, though acral or flexural erythema with dysesthesia is most common and this process is self-limited. Viral exanthem and drug hypersensitivity are the most challenging diagnoses to differentiate from acute cutaneous GVHD. Skin biopsy is commonly requested; unfortunately, this test has poor ability to confirm or exclude GVHD [5–9]. Clinical findings suggestive of GVHD instead of drug hypersensitivity include acral involvement of the face, palms and soles, diarrhea, and hyperbilirubinemia [5, 10]. In a review by Byun et al., a morbilliform rash that was accompanied by diarrhea and hyperbilirubinemia occurred only in the acute GVHD group [10]. In the current case, no skin biopsy was done due to the high clinical suspicion of acute GHVD given cutaneous and hepatic manifestations. In rare cases we will consider skin biopsy, particularly when an alternative diagnosis, such as a cutaneous infection, has distinct histologic findings. We may also consider a skin biopsy if the clinical presentation is atypical; in this situation, the pretest probability for an alternative diagnosis increases.

Treatment Plan

The initial treatment for acute cutaneous GVHD depends on severity; <25 % body surface area (BSA) involvement can be managed with topical corticosteroids and/or topical calcineurin inhibitors (CNI), whereas greater body surface area or any bullous disease requires systemic therapies [4–6]. Topical therapy should be considered as monotherapy for low-grade skin limited acute GVHD, and as adjuvant therapy for acute cutaneous GVHD of any severity or extent of involvement. While high potency topical corticosteroids are generally avoided on the face, major body folds, and genital region, use can be considered for short periods of time in severe cases, particularly with close monitoring. Topical CNI, such as tacrolimus or pimecrolimus, are an excellent alternative in patients who do not improve with topical corticosteroid therapy, and may be most effective when used in combination with topical steroids. Topical CNI provide immunosuppressive benefit equivalent to a class 4 or class 5 topical corticosteroid [11]. However, it is important to note when using a topical CNI, systemic absorption may occur, especially with application to erosions or ulcerations. Thus, serum level monitoring should be considered with extensive or prolonged use [12].

For acute cutaneous GVHD that involves more than 25 % of BSA (stage 2 or higher), systemic corticosteroids at doses of 1–3 mg/kg/day in addition to optimization of preexisting GVHD prophylactic medications are first-line interventions [1–6]. In the presented case, the patient was started on topical corticosteroids (class 3 to the trunk, and a class 5 to the face and genitalia) and methylprednisolone 2 mg/kg/day with improvement over the subsequent 2 weeks. Therapies for more extensive and refractory acute GVHD are discussed in Case 6.2.

Prognosis

Overall patient survival post-allogeneic HSCT is associated with grade of acute GVHD [5, 13]. Gratwohl et al. reported transplant-related mortality for grades 0–4 acute GVHD was 28 %, 27 %, 43 %, 68 %, and 92 %, respectively [13]. In the presented case, the patient had grade 1 acute GVHD confined only to the skin. Unfortunately, this patient passed away about 200 days post-transplant due to disseminated aspergillosis during re-induction chemotherapy for relapsed AML. Development of acute GVHD is also strongly associated with development of chronic GVHD [14]. At the time of passing, the presented patient did not have findings of chronic GVHD.

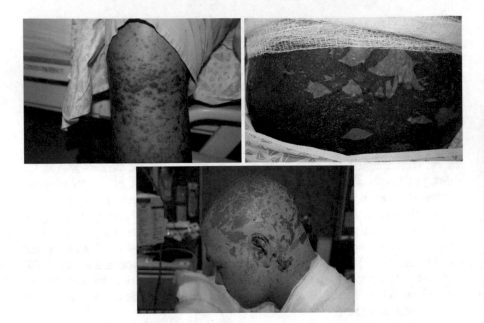

Fig. 6.2 Erythematous and purpuric macules and patches involving 90 % BSA, with multiple denuded areas on the trunk consistent with TEN-like acute GVHD of the skin

Case 6.2

Presentation

A 15-year-old boy who underwent a fully matched unrelated donor bone marrow HSCT for acute lymphoblastic leukemia (ALL) was admitted to the pediatric oncology service 50 days post-transplant due to a quickly evolving full body rash. The rash was initially pruritic and started on the neck and face 4–5 days prior to arrival. On day of admission the patient had erythema involving over 50 % of body surface area (BSA) with new skin discomfort and focal tenderness. He did not have abdominal discomfort, nausea, vomiting, or diarrhea and initially denied involvement of mucosa. He had received prednisone, cyclosporine, and a short course of methotrexate for GVHD prophylaxis.

Physical Exam

On physical examination, the patient appeared ill. He had over 90 % BSA involvement with erythematous and purpuric macules and patches (Fig. 6.2a). Notably, there was desquamation on the trunk, arms, and legs. There were multiple areas on the trunk which were denuded, but without bleeding or ulcerations (Fig. 6.2b). There was xerosis and desquamation of his scalp and face (Fig. 6.2c). There were few erosions and ulcerations on his left lateral epicanthal fold and multiple fingertips. He endorsed diffuse skin tenderness.

Labs

- White blood cells 660 cells/μL (5240–9740 cells/μL)
- Hemoglobin 9.0 (13.5–17.5 g/dL)
- Platelet count 62 billion/L (150–450 billion/L)
- BUN 19 (5–18 mg/dL)
- Creatinine 0.8 mg/dL
- AST 30 unit/L (10–40 μ/L)
- ALT 58 unit/L (7–56 μ/L)
- Total bilirubin 0.2 mg/dL (0.3–1.2 mg/dL)

Questions

1. What are the most likely diagnosis and differential diagnosis?
2. What treatment would you consider?

Discussion

Stage IV, Acute Graft-Versus-Host Disease

The presented patient was clinically diagnosed with stage IV acute cutaneous GVHD based on the International Bone Marrow Transplant Registry (IBMTR) criteria [15]. Due to clinical similarity with toxic epidermal necrolysis (TEN), this presentation is sometimes referred to as TEN-like acute GVHD. Differential diagnosis should include drug-induced TEN or Stevens–Johnson Syndrome (SJS), staphylococcal scalded skin syndrome (SSSS), and toxic shock syndrome (TSS). Full infectious evaluation is a critical first step in any similar case. Subsequent differentiation from drug-induced TEN may be challenging. Based on the single center experience of Goiriz et al., clinical clues that favor stage IV GVHD include gastrointestinal symptoms, elevation of hepatic inflammatory markers, minimal involvement of mucosal sites, and history of pruritus with an exanthem that starts acrally [16]. Skin biopsy is commonly performed when clinical diagnosis is not clear; however, the utility of biopsy in this circumstance remains unclear given similar histologic findings that can be found in both TEN and stage IV, aGVHD. The appropriate diagnosis is paramount as mortality for stage IV acute cutaneous GVHD approaches 90 % compared to about 30 % in TEN. Management of these conditions also differs [16, 17]. In the Goiriz et al. case series, only 2 of 15 patients with TEN-like acute GVHD survived; the most common causes of death were infection and pulmonary GVHD [16]. Fortunately, and as noted in case 1, the incidence of high-grade GVHD has decreased from 30 % to about 8 %, with the introduction of high resolution allele matching [1].

Case Continued and Treatment Considerations

In the presented case, there was no history to suggest a TEN-like drug reaction, and no infectious findings or vital sign abnormalities to suggest SSSS or TSS. The first 6 days of hospital management included an immediate transition to high dose intravenous corticosteroids at a dose of 1 g/m^2, continuation of cyclosporine titrated to therapeutic trough measurements, addition of topical tacrolimus ointment to the face and eyes, and a swish/spit formulation of dexamethasone for oral mucosal involvement. Despite the above interventions, the patient's skin continued to progress with development of duskiness, bullae, and desquamation.

Management of acute GVHD is multifactorial and was briefly discussed in Case 6.1. In 2012, the British Committee for Standards in Haematology developed guidelines to standardize a therapeutic ladder [5]. This committee recommended high dose systemic corticosteroids as first-line therapy. For patients who do not appropriately respond to corticosteroids within 5–7 days, the guidelines suggest addition of a second-line agent. Second-line therapies include mycophenolate mofetil (MMF), anti-tumor necrosis factor (TNF) agents, mammalian target of rapamycin (mTOR) inhibitors, interleukin-2 receptor antibodies, and extracorporeal photopheresis (ECP) [5]. Unfortunately, there has been no definitive evidence to suggest the most effective second-line therapy [5, 18]. Third-line agents include mesenchymal stem cells (MSCs), alemtuzumab, pentostatin, and low dose methotrexate. Lastly, antithymocyte globulin (ATG) and regulatory T cell infusion have been described as novel therapies [5].

In the presented case, the patient was started on ECP after lack of improvement with 6 days of high dose corticosteroids. ECP was administered twice per week, and the patient's corticosteroid dose was slowly tapered. Over the next 3 weeks the patient dramatically improved with a combination of ECP, aggressive wound care, and infection prophylaxis. He was discharged 5 weeks after hospital admission with full reepithelialization. ECP was continued as an outpatient for the next several months.

Extracorporeal photopheresis (ECP) is an attractive option in corticosteroid-refractory acute GVHD due to a favorable side effect profile, as compared to the other second-line therapies. Although the mechanism is poorly understood, it is believed that this therapy induces apoptosis, modulates cytokine production, and expands regulatory T cells [5, 18, 19]. ECP is a well-established therapy in chronic GVHD and studies in adults with steroid-refractory grades II to IV acute GVHD have shown response rates of around 60 % [19, 20]. The side effects of ECP are generally mild with the most serious events related to central catheter-associated thrombosis or infection [19, 20]. In children, hemodynamic monitoring is particularly important as the volume shifts associated with ECP are not adjusted by weight or age. The largest single center series evaluating pediatric use of ECP in steroid-refractory acute GVHD showed a response rate of 72 % [18]. In their case series, 18 % had stage four acute cutaneous GVHD; interestingly, the response to ECP was equivalent regardless of GVHD staging [18]. The dermatology team can play a critical role in the diagnosis of acute GVHD, and as shown in this case, can allow the primary team to quickly initiate potentially lifesaving therapies. Based on our experience and the reviewed literature, ECP is our preferred intervention for severe acute cutaneous GVHD and dermatologists should be aware of this therapeutic option.

Prognosis

Despite successful treatment of acute GVHD, this patient progressed to develop severe cutaneous and pulmonary chronic GVHD leading to a double lung transplant. He subsequently developed respiratory infections and passed away about 2½ years from initial HSCT.

Case 6.3

Presentation

A 5-year-old girl who had a fully matched unrelated bone marrow HSCT 2 years prior for relapsed ALL presented with a bright red, pruritic eruption, which started about 2 weeks prior. Her mom reported that the initial area of involvement was on the face, with subsequent spread to the back and body, along with new scale on the scalp. There was no known preceding illness, sunburn, or new medication exposures. Since the onset of the rash, she endorsed loose stools and hair loss. She denied burning or itching of the eyes, mouth, and genital region. Of note, she had a history of mild acute gastrointestinal GVHD and was weaned off systemic corticosteroids 2 months prior to onset of this eruption. She was not on any other immunosuppressive medications. For this eruption, her oncology team initiated triamcinolone 0.1 % ointment once daily with fluocinolone oil to the scalp, with minimal improvement. On the day of our encounter, the patient and mom endorsed new "skin tightening" in addition to the ongoing red rash.

Physical Exam

On physical examination, the patient was well appearing with a Cushingoid body habitus. She had multiple violaceous scaly oval plaques on the face and trunk with associated hypo- and hyperpigmentation (Fig. 6.3a). Notably, there was subtle

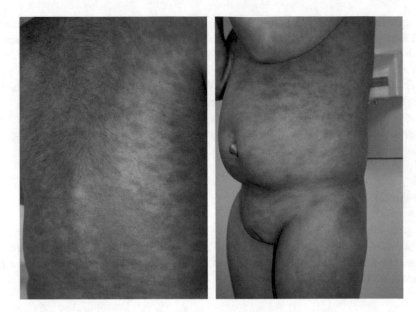

Fig. 6.3 Multiple violaceous scaly oval plaques on the face and trunk and subtle tightening of the skin along the waistband and hips, consistent with early sclerotic chronic GVHD of the skin

tightening and glistening of the skin along the waistband and hips (Fig. 6.3b). She also had protuberance of the mons pubis with erythema and erosions of the labia minora.

Questions

1. What is the patient's diagnosis? What are other morphologies seen in the disease process?
2. What is the treatment plan? What are other novel treatments that can be considered?

Discussion

Chronic Graft-Versus-Host Disease in Children

The presented patient was clinically diagnosed with early cutaneous chronic GVHD (cGVHD), exhibiting lichen planus-like and sclerotic features. Early dermatologic diagnosis of cGVHD ensured quick initiation of systemic therapy by her oncology team as described in detail below. The expected incidence of cGVHD after allogeneic HSCT in children is 20–50%, which is lower than the expected incidence in adults of 60–70% [14, 21]. The median time of cGVHD onset in children is about 6 months [14]. Risk factors for cGVHD are similar to aGVHD with some relevant differences. The source of HSCT is an important factor as recent evidence shows highest rates of cGVHD after peripheral blood HSCT (PBSCT), and lowest rates of cGVHD after matched sibling cord blood HSCT [21–24]. The strongest predictor of chronic GVHD is history of acute GVHD, as noted in Case 6.2 [21]. Other risk factors include HLA mismatch, total body irradiation, splenectomy in the host, and CMV seropositivity in the donor [14]. Like aGVHD, the skin is the most common organ involved in cGVHD.

Based on the National Institute of Health Consensus Development Project classification of cutaneous cGVHD, several findings are diagnostic: poikiloderma, lichen planus-like lesions, lichen sclerosus-like lesions, morphea-like sclerosis, and deep sclerosis [25]. In our experience, true lichen planus-like lesions are rare in children, although patients may present with violaceous patches and plaques that are reminiscent of a lichenoid eruption. Sclerotic cutaneous cGVHD represents a spectrum of phenotypes as a result of fibrosis involving the upper dermis (lichen sclerosus-like plaques), full thickness of the dermis (morphea-like plaques), and/or subcutaneous tissue (deep sclerosis or fasciitis) [21, 25]. Severe sclerotic cGVHD can lead to joint contractures, calcinosis, and poorly healing shallow ulcerations [14, 21]. Other nonsclerotic manifestations of cutaneous cGVHD include ichthyosiform, papulosquamous, psoriasiform, eczematous, and exfoliative lesions. Mucosal findings are common and thus it is critical to carefully examine the eyes, mouth, and genital region [21, 25].

Sclerotic features were subtle in our patient, with lichen sclerosus-like lesions of the inguinal folds, and morphea-like lesions localized to areas of pressure along the waistband. The latter is an example of the isomorphic response seen in sclerotic cGVHD [21, 26]. Similarly, sclerotic cGVHD may be accentuated at other sites of friction or trauma. Thus, in all patients with suspected cutaneous cGVHD, the underwear region should be carefully examined for such findings. Detection of subtle findings may allow for early diagnosis and prompt treatment. The presented patient also exhibited lichen planus-like skin lesions on the face and trunk as well as scarring alopecia. Multiple morphologies may be present in a single patient with cutaneous cGVHD and thus should not deter one away from this diagnosis.

Initial Treatment of Chronic Graft-Versus-Host Disease in Children

In the presented case, initial management included initiation of systemic corticosteroids at a dose of 1 mg/kg/day in addition to topical tacrolimus ointment and high potency topical corticosteroids. Due to ongoing development of sclerotic plaques, extracorporeal photophoresis (ECP) was started 3 weeks later on a twice-weekly regimen, with stabilization of her disease. However, after tapering of prednisone and ECP, she developed new sclerotic plaques and worsening of preexisting lesions. She resumed systemic corticosteroids and was enrolled in a trial of low dose subcutaneous interleukin-2 (IL-2). Eight months later she was fully weaned off systemic corticosteroids while continuing IL-2, with significant improvement.

Treatment of cutaneous cGVHD in children shares some similarities to aGVHD therapy, with data largely based on adult studies. In general, cGVHD therapy is challenging with more than 50 % of patients continuing immunosuppression for more than 2 years [27]. For limited nonsclerotic disease, topical corticosteroids and topical calcineurin inhibitors (CNI) represent first-line therapy [14, 21, 25]. Lichen sclerosus-like lesions may also be responsive to topical therapy. Other forms of sclerotic disease require systemic therapy, which typically starts with corticosteroids at a dose of 1–2 mg/kg/day with or without cyclosporine or tacrolimus [21, 22, 27]. However, topical therapies should also be used adjunctively. For quickly progressive or refractory disease (as in the presented case), multiple second- and third-line options exist (referred to as "salvage therapy"): sirolimus, mycophenolate mofetil, pentostatin, ultraviolet A phototherapy (UVA), narrow band ultraviolet B phototherapy (nbUVB), ECP, rituximab, thalidomide, imatinib mesylate, methotrexate, and other new therapeutics [21, 22, 28]. However, most of these agents have not shown promising results in larger studies.

Of note, UVA and nbUVB are treatment modalities available primarily to the dermatologist and should be considered in select patients with cutaneous cGVHD. A recent multicenter review found improvement in 17/25 patients (all adults) with sclerotic disease, three of whom had complete resolution [29]. Narrow band UVB has shown minimal benefit in sclerotic disease but promising results in lichen planus-like GVHD [30]. A recent pediatric study by Brazzelli et al. showed complete remission of lichen planus-like lesions in 8/10 children after 7 weeks of nbUVB (also treated concurrently with systemic immunosuppression) [31].

Multiple studies of ECP in cutaneous cGVHD have shown favorable clinical responses between 40 and 80 % [32–34]. ECP has not been as effective for cGVHD of other organs such as the gastrointestinal tract. As noted in Case 6.2, ECP is not immunosuppressive and is well tolerated. ECP patients typically receive infusions twice weekly for 12 weeks, and subsequently spaced to every 2 weeks. This time commitment along with the requirement for central line placement may preclude many children from proceeding with therapy. In the presented patient, ECP initially halted progression of sclerotic cGVHD, followed by worsening of disease, prompting therapeutic transition to IL-2. Low dose interleukin-2 therapy is a novel approach that expands T regulatory cell populations and is currently in clinical trials. Koreth et al. showed promising results of low dose IL-2 as a therapeutic option for sclerotic cGVHD in a phase 1 trial and Kennedy-Nasser et al. showed promising results of low dose IL-2 in the prophylaxis of aGVHD [35, 36]. This case demonstrates the critical value of dermatologic care in recognizing early cutaneous cGVHD as well as the importance of understanding the broad array of therapeutic options.

Case 6.4

Presentation

An 18-year-old girl who had a 9/10 HLA-matched unrelated HSCT due to bone marrow failure in setting of dyskeratosis congenita presented to our dermatology clinic for a new rash about 7 months after HSCT. There was no history of acute GVHD. The new rash was pruritic, and started about 1 month prior to evaluation as dry patches on the neck, that subsequently spread to involve the face, scalp, trunk, and extremities. She denied blisters, or involvement of mucosal surfaces. The rash was not preceded by infectious symptoms or new medications, though her dose of cyclosporine was decreased about 2 weeks prior to onset of rash. Initial evaluation by the oncology team resulted in diagnosis of xerosis due to dry winter weather. Prior therapies included multiple emollients without any improvement.

Physical Exam

On physical examination, the patient appeared well nourished in no acute distress. There was generalized and prominent xerosis involving her face, scalp, trunk, and extremities (Fig. 6.4a). There was ichthyosiform scale on the trunk and extremities, most prominently on the back and buttocks (Fig. 6.4b). Xerosis was accentuated around follicles. There were superficial fissures and scaly plaques on the dorsal hands, anterior thighs, and ankles. There was prominent hypopigmentation underlying areas of involvement. The scalp had prominent scale with generalized thinning of the hair. Subtle ectropion was noted bilaterally. The nails, mouth, and genitalia were normal. There were no blisters noted on exam.

Labs

- AST: 19 (10–40 IU/L)
- ALT: 33 (7–56 IU/L)
- Albumin: 4.2 (3–6 IU/L)
- WBC: 6.7 billion cells/L (3.5–10.5 billion cells/L)
- HBG: 11.2 g/dL (12.0–15.5 g/dL)

Clinical Questions

1. What is the diagnosis?
2. What is the prognosis for ichthyosiform cGVHD of the skin?
3. What is the management ladder for this patient?

Fig. 6.4 Generalized and
prominent xerosis
involving her scalp, face,
trunk, and extremities with
ichthyosiform scaling on
the trunk and extremities,
consistent with
ichthyosiform chronic
GVHD of the skin

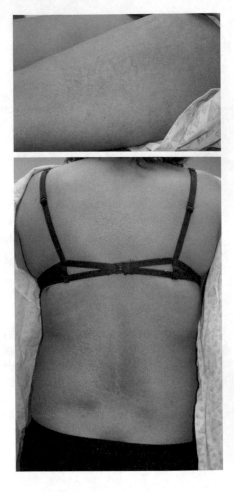

Discussion

Ichthyosiform Cutaneous Chronic GVHD

This patient was diagnosed with ichthyosiform cutaneous cGVHD, a nonsclerotic
type of cGVHD. Clinical clues to diagnosis included sudden and rapidly progressive onset in a patient without prior history of ichthyosis, follicular involvement,
and associated alopecia. In addition, profound dyspigmentation is commonly
encountered in this variant of cutaneous cGVHD. Risk factors for cGVHD are
reviewed in Case 6.3. Of mention, the use of alemtuzumab in this patient's conditioning regimen served as a T-cell depleting agent, which may have served a protective role against severe cGVHD. Chakrabarthi showed that adult patients treated
with alemtuzumab before allogeneic stem cell transplant had significantly decreased
rates of cGVHD [37].

Nonsclerotic phenotypes represent up to 80 % of cutaneous cGVHD cases [14, 21, 38–40]. Of note, the historical term "lichenoid" cutaneous cGVHD was applied to all nonsclerotic phenotypes, though we recommend this term be reserved for histologically defined disease given the wide spectrum of nonsclerotic cutaneous cGVHD. In adults, the most common nonsclerotic phenotypes include lichen planus-like lesions, poikilodermatous (combination of atrophy, telangiectasia, and pigmentary changes to the skin), and erythematous maculopapular lesions [21, 38–40]. Ichthyosiform and eczematous variants of cutaneous cGVHD have been reported rarely in adults, but may be more prevalent in children [40–42]. In our experience, children with these forms of cGVHD are less likely to have visceral involvement and have a better prognosis than those with sclerotic cGVHD [41]. In adults, only a minority of patients with nonsclerotic cutaneous cGVHD progress to develop sclerotic features [39, 40].

Skin Biopsy Consideration, Therapeutic Plan, and Clinical Course Continued

Based on the NIH consensus guidelines, clinical findings that are diagnostic for cutaneous cGVHD and do not require biopsy include poikiloderma, lichen planus-like lesions, lichen sclerosus-like lesions, morphea-like sclerosis, and deep sclerosis [25]. Skin biopsy can be considered in atypical forms of cutaneous cGVHD, and may show interface dermatitis with vacuolar changes, and a sparse to dense lichenoid infiltrate. Presence of periadnexal inflammation would favor the diagnosis of cGVHD [43]. In the presented case, a skin biopsy was offered to the family, who opted to pursue a therapeutic trial instead.

As discussed in detail in Case 6.3, the therapeutic ladder for cutaneous cGVHD consists of topical immunosuppressive agents for limited nonsclerotic cutaneous disease, and systemic therapy for more extensive or sclerotic cutaneous disease [4, 27]. We present our approach to successful topical therapy for nonsclerotic cutaneous cGVHD.

At the first visit, the patient was started on a combination of topical corticosteroids including triamcinolone 0.1 % ointment to the face and flexural areas, clobetasol 0.05 % ointment to the most active areas excluding the face/flexures, and fluocinolone oil for the scalp. Prior emollients were discontinued, and instead hydrated petrolatum was started and applied twice daily on top of the topical steroids. Occlusion with plastic (Saran) wrap was utilized to improve cutaneous absorption, in areas where this was possible (trunk, arms, legs, hands, neck). At follow-up visit 2 weeks later, the skin of her face, trunk, and extremities was almost fully clear, with residual light brown hyperpigmentation in areas of prior thick scale. Based on this response, skin biopsy was unnecessary. At that visit the patient stepped down from clobetasol to triamcinolone 0.1 % ointment to any affected area for no more than 2 weeks continuously in addition to twice daily hydrated petrolatum to the entire body and continued on fluocinolone 0.01 % oil to the scalp. Over the subsequent 8 months we evaluated the patient about once per month and she developed intermittent mild flares of eczematous and ichthyotic plaques, with one episode of a lichen sclerosus-like plaque. All of these flares responded to 1–2 weeks of clobetasol 0.05 % ointment under occlusion, followed by every other day triamcinolone 0.1 % ointment until full resolution. While erythema and scaling of her scalp improved, she had persistent hair thinning that gradually improved over the course of 1 year with intermittent use of topical corticosteroids and minoxidil 5 % solution. She never developed cGVHD of any other organ system, and never required systemic immunosuppression to treat cutaneous cGVHD. The patient is now 3 years post-HSCT and off all systemic immunosuppression, without significant complications arising from therapy.

Nonsclerotic cutaneous cGVHD is a disease with protean manifestations, and a good prognosis. It is critical for dermatologists to recognize the wide spectrum of this disease, and intervene early to prevent morbidity.

References

1. Jacobsohn DA. Acute graft-versus-host disease in children. Bone Marrow Transplant. 2008;41(2):215–21.
2. Eisner MD, August CS. Impact of donor and recipient characteristics on the development of acute and chronic graft-versus-host disease following pediatric bone marrow transplantation. Bone Marrow Transplant. 1995;15(5):663–8.
3. Filipovich AH, Weisdorf D, Pavletic S, Socie G, Wingard JR, Lee SJ, et al. National Institutes of Health consensus development project on criteria for clinical trials in chronic graft-versus-host disease: I. Diagnosis and staging working group report. Biol Blood Marrow Transplant. 2005;11:945–56.
4. Hymes SR, Alousi AM, Cowen EW. Graft-versus-host disease: part II. Management of cutaneous graft-versus-host disease. J Am Acad Dermatol. 2012;66(4):535.e1–16.
5. Dignan FL, Clark A, Amrolia P, et al. Diagnosis and management of acute graft-versus-host disease. Br J Haematol. 2012;158(1):30–45.
6. Hu SW, Cotliar J. Acute graft-versus-host disease following hematopoietic stem-cell transplantation. Dermatol Ther. 2011;24(4):411–23.
7. Firoz BF, Lee SJ, Nghiem P, Qureshi AA. Role of skin biopsy to confirm suspected acute graft-vs-host disease: results of decision analysis. Arch Dermatol. 2006;142(2):175–82.
8. Kuykendall TD, Smoller BR. Lack of specificity in skin biopsy specimens to assess for acute graft-versus-host disease in initial 3 weeks after bone-marrow transplantation. J Am Acad Dermatol. 2003;49(6):1081–5.
9. Zhou Y, Barnett MJ, Rivers JK. Clinical significance of skin biopsies in the diagnosis and management of graft-vs-host disease in early postallogeneic bone marrow transplantation. Arch Dermatol. 2000;136(6):717–21.
10. Byun HJ, Yang JI, Kim BK, Cho KH. Clinical differentiation of acute cutaneous graft-versus-host disease from drug hypersensitivity reactions. J Am Acad Dermatol. 2011;65(4):726–32.
11. Frankel HC, Qureshi AA. Comparative effectiveness of topical calcineurin inhibitors in adult patients with atopic dermatitis. Am J Clin Dermatol. 2012;13(2):113–23.
12. Olson KA, West K, Mccarthy PL. Toxic tacrolimus levels after application of topical tacrolimus and use of occlusive dressings in two bone marrow transplant recipients with cutaneous graft-versus-host disease. Pharmacotherapy. 2014;34(6):e60–4.

13. Gratwohl A, Hermans J, Apperley J, et al. Acute graft-versus-host disease: grade and outcome in patients with chronic myelogenous leukemia. Working Party Chronic Leukemia of the European Group for Blood and Marrow Transplantation. Blood. 1995;86(2):813–8.

14. Baird K, Cooke K, Schultz KR. Chronic graft-versus-host disease (GVHD) in children. Pediatr Clin North Am. 2010;57(1):297–322.

15. Rowlings PA, Przepiorka D, Klein JP, et al. IBMTR Severity Index for grading acute graft-versus-host disease: retrospective comparison with Glucksberg grade. Br J Haematol. 1997;97(4):855–64.

16. Goiriz R, Peñas P, Pérez-gala S, et al. Stage IV cutaneous acute graft-versus-host disease. Clinical and histological study of 15 cases. J Eur Acad Dermatol Venereol. 2009;23(12):1398–404.

17. Irvine AD, Hoeger PH, Yan AC. Harper's textbook of pediatric dermatology. West Sussex: Wiley-Blackwell; 2011.

18. Calore E, Marson P, Pillon M, et al. Treatment of acute graft-versus-host disease in childhood with extracorporeal photochemotherapy/photopheresis: the Padova experience. Biol Blood Marrow Transplant. 2015;21(11):1963–72.

19. Couriel D, Hosing C, Saliba R, et al. Extracorporeal photopheresis for acute and chronic graft-versus-host disease: does it work? Biol Blood Marrow Transplant. 2006;12(1 Suppl 2):37–40.

20. Abu-dalle I, Reljic T, Nishihori T, et al. Extracorporeal photopheresis in steroid-refractory acute or chronic graft-versus-host disease: results of a systematic review of prospective studies. Biol Blood Marrow Transplant. 2014;20(11):1677–86.

21. Hymes SR, Alousi AM, Cowen EW. Graft-versus-host disease: part I. Pathogenesis and clinical manifestations of graft-versus-host disease. J Am Acad Dermatol. 2012;66(4):515.e1–18.

22. Holtick U, Albrecht M, Chemnitz JM, et al. Bone marrow versus peripheral blood allogeneic haematopoietic stem cell transplantation for haematological malignancies in adults. Cochrane Database Syst Rev. 2014;4:CD010189.

23. Rocha V, Wagner JE, Sobocinski KA, et al. Graft-versus-host disease in children who have received a cord-blood or bone marrow transplant from an HLA-identical sibling. Eurocord and International Bone Marrow Transplant Registry Working Committee on Alternative Donor and Stem Cell Sources. N Engl J Med. 2000;342(25):1846–54.

24. Wagner JE, Kernan NA, Steinbuch M, Broxmeyer HE, Gluckman E. Allogeneic sibling umbilical-cord-blood transplantation in children with malignant and non-malignant disease. Lancet. 1995;346(8969):214–9.

25. Jagasia MH, Greinix HT, Arora M, et al. National institutes of health consensus development project on criteria for clinical trials in chronic graft-versus-host disease: I. The 2014 diagnosis and staging working group report. Biol Blood Marrow Transplant. 2015;21(3):389–401.e1.

26. Patel AR, Pavletic SZ, Turner ML, Cowen EW. The isomorphic response in morphea-like chronic graft-vs-host disease. Arch Dermatol. 2008;144(9):1229–31.

27. Arora M. Therapy of chronic graft-versus-host disease. Best Pract Res Clin Haematol. 2008;21(2):271–9.

28. Wolff D, Schleuning M, Von harsdorf S, et al. Consensus conference on clinical practice in chronic GVHD: second-line treatment of chronic graft-versus-host disease. Biol Blood Marrow Transplant. 2011;17(1):1–17.

29. Connolly KL, Griffith JL, Mcevoy M, Lim HW. Ultraviolet A1 phototherapy beyond morphea: experience in 83 patients. Photodermatol Photoimmunol Photomed. 2015;31(6):289–95.

30. Enk CD, Elad S, Vexler A, Kapelushnik J, Gorodetsky R, Kirschbaum M. Chronic graft-versus-host disease treated with UVB phototherapy. Bone Marrow Transplant. 1998;22(12):1179–83.

31. Brazzelli V, Grasso V, Muzio F, et al. Narrowband ultraviolet B phototherapy in the treatment of cutaneous graft-versus-host disease in oncohaematological paediatric patients. Br J Dermatol. 2010;162(2):404–9.

32. Apisarnthanarax N, Donato M, Körbling M, et al. Extracorporeal photopheresis therapy in the management of steroid-refractory or steroid-dependent cutaneous chronic graft-versus-host disease after allogeneic stem cell transplantation: feasibility and results. Bone Marrow Transplant. 2003;31(6):459–65.

33. Foss FM, Divenuti GM, Chin K, et al. Prospective study of extracorporeal photopheresis in steroid-refractory or steroid-resistant extensive chronic graft-versus-host disease: analysis of response and survival incorporating prognostic factors. Bone Marrow Transplant. 2005;35(12):1187–93.

34. Greinix HT, Volc-platzer B, Rabitsch W, et al. Successful use of extracorporeal photochemo-therapy in the treatment of severe acute and chronic graft-versus-host disease. Blood. 1998;92(9):3098–104.

35. Kennedy-nasser AA, Ku S, Castillo-caro P, et al. Ultra low-dose IL-2 for GVHD prophylaxis after allogeneic hematopoietic stem cell transplantation mediates expansion of regulatory T cells without diminishing antiviral and antileukemic activity. Clin Cancer Res. 2014;20(8):2215–25.

36. Koreth J, Matsuoka K, Kim HT, et al. Interleukin-2 and regulatory T cells in graft-versus-host disease. N Engl J Med. 2011;365(22):2055–66.

37. Chakrabarti S, MacDonald D, Hale G, Holder K, Turner V, Czarnecka H, Thompson J, Fegan C, Waldmann H, Milligan DW. T-cell depletion with Campath-1H "in the bag" for matched related allogeneic peripheral blood stem cell transplantation is associated with reduced graft-versus-host disease, rapid immune constitution and improved survival. Br J Haematol. 2003;121:109–18.

38. Chosidow O, Bagot M, Vernant JP, Roujeau JC, Cordonnier C, Kuentz M, et al. Sclerodermatous chronic graft-versus-host disease. Analysis of seven cases. J Am Acad Dermatol. 1992;26:49–55.

39. Skert C, Patriarca F, Sperotto A, Cerno M, Fili C, Zaja F, et al. Sclerodermatous chronic graft-versus-host disease after allogeneic hematopoietic stem cell transplantation: incidence, predictors and outcome. Haematologica. 2006;91:258–61.

40. Kim SJ, Choi JM, Kim JE, Cho BK, Kim DW, Park HJ. Clinicopathologic characteristics of cutaneous chronic graft-versus-host diseases: a retrospective study in Korean patients. Int J Dermatol. 2010;49(12):1386–92.

41. Huang JT, Duncan CN, Boyer D, Khosravi H, Lehmann LE, Saavedra A. Nail dystrophy, edema, and eosinophilia: harbingers of severe chronic GVHD of the skin in children. Bone Marrow Transplant. 2014;49(12):1521–7.

42. Creamer D, Martyn-simmons CL, Osborne G, et al. Eczematoid graft-vs-host disease: a novel form of chronic cutaneous graft-vs-host disease and its response to psoralen UV-A therapy. Arch Dermatol. 2007;143(9):1157–62.

43. Shulman HM, Cardona DM, Greenson JK, et al. NIH Consensus development project on criteria for clinical trials in chronic graft-versus-host disease: II. The 2014 Pathology Working Group Report. Biol Blood Marrow Transplant. 2015;21(4):589–603.

Chapter 7
Autoimmune Skin Disorders (Collagen Vascular)

Clayton Sontheimer and Heather A. Brandling-Bennett

Abstract Autoimmune connective tissue diseases are frequently in the differential diagnosis when patients present with cutaneous eruptions and systemic complaints. Systemic-onset juvenile idiopathic arthritis, systemic lupus erythematosus, and juvenile dermatomyositis are three autoimmune disorders that may have prominent cutaneous findings. Recognition of the characteristic skin manifestations may be critical in ordering the appropriate workup and making the correct diagnosis.

Keywords Autoimmune • Systemic-onset juvenile idiopathic arthritis • Still's disease • Systemic lupus erythematosus • Juvenile dermatomyositis

Case 7.1

History

You are asked to see a 4-year-old boy who was admitted for fevers of unknown origin. Three weeks ago, he began having spiking fevers up to 104 F every day. The fevers initially occurred at any time of the day but recently occur only in the late afternoon. During fever spikes, he has chills, joint pain, and a pink-red rash over his trunk and arms. The joint pain and rash improve after his temperature returns to normal. In between fever spikes, he feels well though his parents note that he seems to be walking differently.

C. Sontheimer, MD
Division of Rheumatology, Department of Pediatrics,
Seattle Children's Hospital/University of Washington, Seattle, WA, USA

H.A. Brandling-Bennett, MD (✉)
Division of Dermatology, Department of Pediatrics, Seattle Children's Hospital/University of Washington, OC.9.835, PO Box 5371, Seattle, WA 98105, USA
e-mail: Heather.Brandling-Bennett@seattlechildrens.org

© Springer International Publishing Switzerland 2016
M. Hogeling (ed.), *Case-Based Inpatient Pediatric Dermatology*,
DOI 10.1007/978-3-319-31569-0_7

Physical Exam

- Vital signs: T 39.2 C (102.9 F), HR 127, RR 20, BP 105/65.
- Skin exam reveals salmon-pink coalescing macules and papules on the trunk with linear lesions demonstrating Koebner phenomenon (Fig. 7.1).
- He has similar lesions on his legs (Fig. 7.2).
- Small, symmetric, shotty lymph nodes are palpable in cervical chains.
- Joint exam shows warm, swollen knees with pain on range of motion.

Labs

- WBC 25.8 (6.0–15.5 K/mm^3)
- HCT: 31.5 (34.0–40 %)
- Platelets: 625 (250–550 K/mm^3)
- CRP 15.8 (nml <0.8 mg/dL)
- ESR 87 (0–10 mm/h)
- Fibrinogen 662 (230–450 mg/dL)
- Ferritin 770 (0–60 ng/mL)
- LDH 781 (425–975 IU/L)
- Uric acid 2.3 (2.0–6.0 mg/dL)
- Infectious workup including blood cultures and viral studies negative

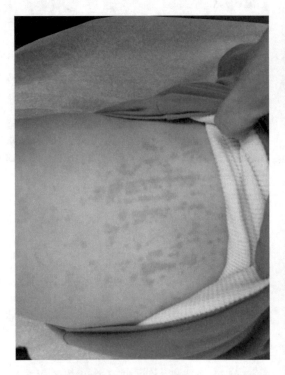

Fig. 7.1 Salmon-pink coalescing macules and papules on the trunk with linear lesions demonstrating Koebner phenomenon

Fig. 7.2 Salmon-pink coalescing macules and papules on the leg

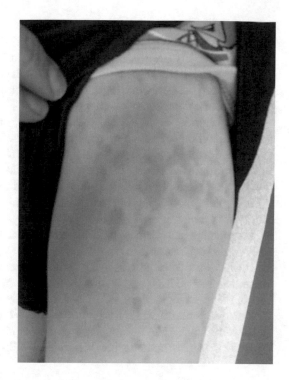

Questions

1. What is the likely diagnosis?
2. What further workup and treatment(s) should be considered?
3. The patient's clinical picture worsens with now persistent fevers, a new petechial rash, and plummeting WBC and platelet levels. What complication should be considered?

Answers

Systemic-onset juvenile idiopathic arthritis (soJIA) represents a small subset of juvenile arthritis (10 % of JIA cases) but is the most frequently encountered subset in the inpatient setting due to the high, spiking fevers and often impressive systemic manifestations. A similar presentation in patients older than 16 years of age is referred to as adult Still's disease. The International League Against Rheumatism (ILAR) criteria for diagnosis of soJIA requires the presence of arthritis, fever >38.5 °C for at least 2 weeks (quotidian for at least 3 days), and one of four additional criteria: hepatosplenomegaly, generalized lymphadenopathy, serositis, and/or evanescent rash. The rash consists of small (usually <5 mm) salmon-pink macules predominantly over the trunk and proximal extremities. The eruption appears during fever spikes and quickly fades after fevers resolve. While not typically pruritic, it can be intensely pruritic in some patients, and koebnerization may be a clue to diagnosis. Diagnosis can be challenging due to the transient nature of the fevers and rash as well as because objective arthritis may not be appreciated early in the course when systemic manifestations are prominent.

The differential diagnosis includes infections, malignancy such as lymphoma or leukemia, and other rheumatologic etiologies like Kawasaki disease. Compared to other diagnostic considerations, patients with soJIA are often strikingly well appearing in between fever spikes. Oncology and infectious disease services, in addition to rheumatology, are often involved in workup and diagnosis. A thorough evaluation for malignancy consisting of chest, abdomen, and pelvis imaging and bone marrow biopsy are often indicated to rule out malignancy.

Macrophage-activation syndrome (MAS) is a life-threatening complication of soJIA, and occurs on the spectrum with the systemic features of soJIA [1]. Macrophage-activation shares many features in common with hemophagocytic lymphohistiocytosis (HLH) and is thought to represent the same pathophysiologic process in rheumatologic diseases [2]. MAS is characterized by persistent high fevers and rash, cytopenias, elevated ferritin levels (often >2000 ng/mL), hypertriglyceridemia, and low fibrinogen. MAS secondary to soJIA requires less aggressive treatment than HLH and is usually treated with IV steroids and IL-1 inhibitors.

Treatment

Treatment of soJIA has advanced significantly in recent years owing to cytokine-specific inhibition of key inflammatory mediators IL-1 and IL-6 [3–6]. IL-1 is central to the systemic inflammation of soJIA, and inhibition of IL-1 with anakinra or canakinumab is very effective in patients who present with fevers. IL-6 inhibition with tocilizumab may be most useful for patients with arthritis and minimal systemic manifestations. Corticosteroids, either IV or PO, are often used as a short-term adjunct therapy, especially in hospitalized patients. Historically, medicines such as methotrexate, cyclosporine, and indomethacin were commonly used but have been replaced by cytokine-specific biologics.

Case 7.2

History

A 14-year-old female presents with a 6-week history of worsening joint pain, fatigue, and rash. Six weeks ago, she developed joint pain in her hands, wrists, and knees that is worse in the morning. Her energy level is decreasing, and she is now tired most of the day. Within the last week, she developed intermittent fevers to 101.5 and a new rash over her hands and cheeks. She also reports a 10 lb weight loss over the past month.

Physical Exam

- Vital Signs: T 37.0, HR 85, RR 20, BP 136/71 (normal 90–130/65–83).
- Skin exam reveals an erythematous malar rash (Fig. 7.3) and erythematous patches on her dorsal hands (Fig. 7.4). Nail fold capillaries appear normal.
- Joint exam demonstrates swelling and warmth to bilateral knees and wrists.

Laboratory Results

- WBC 2.4 (5.0–11.0 K/mm^3)
- ALC 480 (1100–4500/mm^3)
- Hct 20.6 (36.0–46.0%)
- Platelets 147 (150–450 K/mm^3)
- CRP <0.8 (nml <0.8)
- ESR 97 (0–20 mm/h)
- Albumin 2.4 (3.8–5.4 g/dL)
- PTT 36 (25–35 s)
- UA: 3+ blood, 2+ protein
- C3 43 (83–203 mg/dL)
- C4 <7 (15–52 mg/dL)
- Antinuclear antibody screen (ANA): positive, titer 1:640, speckled/homogenous
- Antibodies: positive for anti-dsDNA, anti-Ro/SSA, anti-La/SSB, anti-Smith

Questions

1. What is the most likely diagnosis?
2. What further workup is indicated to help guide treatment decisions?

Answers

The patient presents with multisystem disease and laboratory testing consistent with systemic lupus erythematosus (SLE). The presence of a malar rash in the setting of cytopenias in multiple cell lines, positive ANA, and lupus-specific autoantibodies (anti-dsDNA,

Fig. 7.3 Erythematous
malar rash

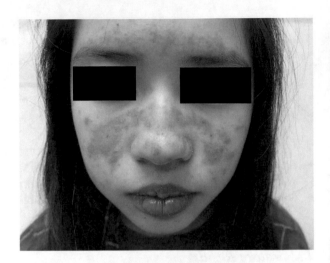

Fig. 7.4 Ill-defined
erythematous patches on
the dorsal hands

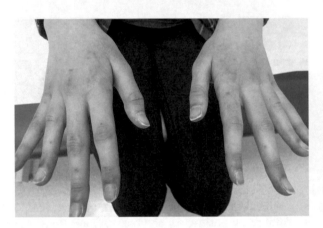

anti-Smith) is highly consistent with SLE and sufficient to meet diagnostic criteria. Though not diagnostic, additional features such low C3/C4 and strikingly elevated ESR with normal-to-mildly elevated CRP are also characteristic of SLE. Diagnosis of SLE is achieved by meeting at least 4 of 11 diagnostic criteria according to the American College of Rheumatology 1997 criteria. More recently, the use of the Systemic Lupus International Collaborating Clinic (SLICC) criteria proposed by Petri et al. [7] has replaced the use of ACR criteria in adults, though the criteria have not been independently validated in children and are not yet widely used in pediatric lupus.

SLE in children can cause a spectrum of cutaneous manifestations similar to that seen in adults, with a few notable differences. Isolated cutaneous disease consisting of either discoid lupus or subacute cutaneous lupus is much less common in children, thus children presenting with cutaneous lupus should be evaluated thoroughly for signs of systemic disease [8]. Similarly, the risk of progression from isolated skin disease to systemic disease may be higher in children than adults. Subacute cutaneous lupus is very rare in pediatrics patients. This is perhaps owing to the fact that children are uncommonly treated with medicines reported to cause drug-induced lupus with the notable exception of minocycline.

The presence of hypertension, hematuria, and proteinuria in the above patient suggests the possibility of lupus nephritis and warrant further investigation to assess the extent of disease. Quantitative measurement of proteinuria (spot protein:creatinine ratio or 24 h urine collection) and kidney biopsy are indicated. Patients with significant nephritis are treated aggressively by induction therapy with either cyclophosphamide or mycophenolate.

Treatment

For patients with systemic disease, systemic corticosteroid therapy (PO and/or IV) is important in inducing remission though should be tapered to the lowest possible therapeutic dose to avoid long-term side effects such as growth failure and osteopenia. Hydroxychloroquine is used in almost all children with SLE, even in those with minimal or absent skin findings. Additional therapy is guided by the extent and severity of disease, or other complications such as MAS. As mentioned above, patients with significant nephritis are commonly treated with cyclophosphamide or mycophenolate. In patients with less severe disease, methotrexate and azathioprine are often used as maintenance therapy. Topical or intralesional corticosteroids and topical calcineurin inhibitors can be used as adjunctive treatment for cutaneous lesions. SLE is a photosensitive condition, and thus counseling regarding photoprotection is important.

Case 7.3

History

You are asked to see a 5-year-old boy with a 2-month history of progressive energy loss, weakness, and rash who was admitted for concerns for aspiration risk. His rash started on his hands and subsequently spread to his feet, elbows, and knees. His energy level has progressively decreased and he tires after minimal activity. Within the past week, he has difficulty with feeding, takes longer to eat, and occasionally coughs with liquids. His parents also think that his voice sounds more nasal than usual.

Physical Exam

Vital signs: T 36.6, HR 86, BP 106/68.

Skin exam reveals coalescing erythematous papules over the dorsal MCP, DIP, and PIP joints (Fig. 7.5) and extensor elbows (Fig. 7.6). Patient also has poorly demarcated confluent erythema surrounding eyelids, cheeks, and nasal bridge. Nailfold capillaries are dilated and tortuous.

Fig. 7.5 Coalescing erythematous papules over the dorsal MCP, DIP, and PIP joints consistent with Gottron's papules

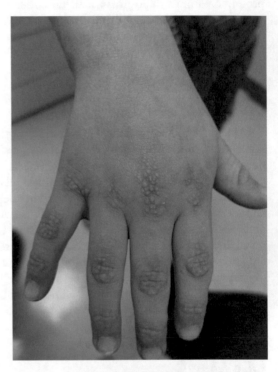

Fig. 7.6 Coalescing erythematous papules over the extensor elbows

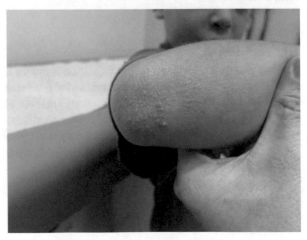

Strength exam shows 3/5 strength in neck flexors, shoulder and hip girdle musculature and 4/5 in distal extremity muscles. Gowers sign is present.

Laboratory Results

- WBC: 10.2 (5.0–13.5 K/mm^3)
- Hct 29.8 (34.0–40 %)
- Platelets 391 (250–550 K/mm^3)
- ESR 44 (0–19 mm/h)
- CRP <0.8 (<0.8 mg/dL)
- BUN 15 (6–20 mg/dL)
- Creatinine 0.2 (0.1–0.6 mg/dL)
- AST 82 (5–41 IU/L)
- ALT 62 (6–40 IU/L)
- Creatine kinase 272 (35–230 IU/L)
- Lactate dehydrogenase 1473 (370–840 IU/L)
- Aldolase 9 (1–7 units/L)
- ANA positive, 1:160 (speckled pattern)

Questions

1. What further testing would confirm the diagnosis?
2. What treatments should be considered?

Answers

The patient presents with classic features of juvenile dermatomyositis (JDM) including Gottron's papules (erythematous papules over the knuckles), nail fold capillary changes, and muscle weakness. Laboratory testing shows elevation in muscle markers (CK, AST, ALT, LDH, and aldolase) and signs of systemic inflammation (elevated ESR and anemia of chronic disease). In this patient, the abnormal swallowing symptoms and voice changes indicate weakness in pharyngeal muscles suggesting advanced disease and put the patient at risk for aspiration. In contrast to adults, JDM is not associated with increased risk of malignancy. Interstitial lung disease is much less common in children, but can occur.

The cutaneous manifestations of JDM are similar to those seen in adults, and patients can present with Gottron's papules or Gottron's sign (erythematous macules and patches over knuckles, elbows, and knees), heliotrope rash (violaceous erythema on upper eyelids, often associated with edema), malar or more extensive facial rash, and nail fold capillary changes (dilatation, tortuosity, and dropout). Erythema or poikiloderma over the shoulders and upper back (shawl sign) or central chest (V-sign) may also be seen. Amyopathic DM can occur but is much less common than in adults [9], thus any child presenting with cutaneous findings of JDM warrants a thorough evaluation for myositis, especially as muscle weakness may be underappreciated. In younger children, myositis may present as irritability or decreased activity before muscle weakness is identified. Calcinosis or dystrophic calcification is more common in JDM than in adults and can occur later in the disease course [10]. It can occur without other skin or muscle symptoms, is difficult to treat and can cause significant morbidity, but is less common with earlier and more aggressive treatment. Cutaneous ulcerations are also more frequent in JDM, typically occurring over areas of calcification or joints.

Historically, electromyography studies or muscle biopsy showing inflammation, perifascicular atrophy, or degeneration/regeneration was performed to confirm diagnosis. More recently, MRI with STIR (short tau inversion recovery) sequence is commonly performed to confirm muscle inflammation as it is readily available, gives faster results, and is less invasive [11].

In general, children with JDM are treated more aggressively than adults. In addition to IV and/or PO corticosteroids, methotrexate and IVIG are commonly started in new patients with JDM. For severe or refractory cases, cyclophosphamide or rituximab (an anti-CD20 monoclonal antibody) are sometimes used. Topical corticosteroids and calcineurin inhibitors may be used as adjunctive treatment for recalcitrant skin disease. Ultraviolet light exposure can exacerbate skin involvement; therefore patients with JDM should be counseled regarding photoprotection.

References

1. Sawhney S, Woo P, Murray KJ. Macrophage activation syndrome: a potentially fatal complication of rheumatic disorders. Arch Dis Child. 2001;85(5):421–6. Epub 2001/10/23.
2. Stephan JL, Kone-Paut I, Galambrun C, Mouy R, Bader-Meunier B, Prieur AM. Reactive haemophagocytic syndrome in children with inflammatory disorders. A retrospective study of 24 patients. Rheumatology. 2001;40(11):1285–92. Epub 2001/11/16.
3. Zeft A, Hollister R, LaFleur B, Sampath P, Soep J, McNally B, et al. Anakinra for systemic juvenile arthritis: the Rocky Mountain experience. J Clin Rheumatol. 2009;15(4):161–4. Epub 2009/04/14.
4. Lequerre T, Quartier P, Rosellini D, Alaoui F, De Bandt M, Mejjad O, et al. Interleukin-1 receptor antagonist (anakinra) treatment in patients with systemic-onset juvenile idiopathic arthritis or adult onset Still disease: preliminary experience in France. Ann Rheum Dis. 2008;67(3):302–8. Epub 2007/10/20.
5. Yokota S, Imagawa T, Mori M, Miyamae T, Aihara Y, Takei S, et al. Efficacy and safety of tocilizumab in patients with systemic-onset juvenile idiopathic arthritis: a randomised, double-blind, placebo-controlled, withdrawal phase III trial. Lancet. 2008;371(9617):998–1006. Epub 2008/03/25.
6. De Benedetti F, Brunner HI, Ruperto N, Kenwright A, Wright S, Calvo I, et al. Randomized trial of tocilizumab in systemic juvenile idiopathic arthritis. N Engl J Med. 2012;367(25):2385–95. Epub 2012/12/21.

7. Petri M, Orbai AM, Alarcon GS, Gordon C, Merrill JT, Fortin PR, et al. Derivation and validation of the Systemic Lupus International Collaborating Clinics classification criteria for systemic lupus erythematosus. Arthritis Rheum. 2012;64(8):2677–86. Epub 2012/05/04.
8. Mina R, Brunner HI. Pediatric lupus—are there differences in presentation, genetics, response to therapy, and damage accrual compared with adult lupus? Rheum Dis Clin North Am. 2010;36(1):53–80, vii–viii. Epub 2010/03/06.
9. Gerami P, Walling HW, Lewis J, Doughty L, Sontheimer RD. A systematic review of juvenile-onset clinically amyopathic dermatomyositis. Br J Dermatol. 2007;157(4):637–44. Epub 2007/06/29.
10. Sallum AM, Pivato FC, Doria-Filho U, Aikawa NE, Liphaus BL, Marie SK, et al. Risk factors associated with calcinosis of juvenile dermatomyositis. J Pediatr. 2008;84(1):68–74. Epub 2008/01/11.
11. Tomasova Studynkova J, Charvat F, Jarosova K, Vencovsky J. The role of MRI in the assessment of polymyositis and dermatomyositis. Rheumatology. 2007;46(7):1174–9. Epub 2007/05/15.

Chapter 8
Inpatient Neonatal Dermatology

Kimberly Jablon and Erin Mathes

Abstract This chapter discusses five cutaneous conditions seen in the newborn period that have implications for the health of the newborn: subcutaneous fat necrosis of the newborn, aplasia cutis, congenital melanocytic nevus, neonatal lupus, and incontinentia pigmenti. Neonatal subcutaneous fat necrosis is a disorder that presents with erythematous nodules in the newborn. It is a self-resolving condition associated with neonatal stress or hypothermia, and may be complicated by hypercalcemia. Aplasia cutis congenita is a heterogeneous group of disorders with many genetic and environmental causes, which all present with absence of the epidermis, and sometimes deeper tissues. Most lesions heal spontaneously with standard wound care, although larger lesions may need to be treated surgically. Neonatal lupus is a transient, passively acquired immune disorder due to maternal antibodies that can affect the skin, heart, and blood. The most serious risk is congenital heart block, which can be permanent and must be screened for carefully. Giant congenital melanocytic nevi are benign proliferations of melanocytes that may be associated with neurocutaneous melanocytosis and malignant melanoma. Proper surveillance for complications and avoidance of unnecessary prophylactic treatment is crucial. Incontinentia pigmenti is a rare dominant X-linked genetic disorder that presents with four distinct stages of skin lesions following the lines of Blaschko. Other systems that may be affected include the central nervous, dental, and ophthalmologic systems.

Keywords Neonatal subcutaneous fat necrosis • Neonatal lupus • Anti-Ro/La antibodies • Lines of Blaschko • Incontinentia pigmenti • Melanocytic nevus • Cutis aplasia • Hypercalcemia • Neurocutaneous melanosis • Congenital heart block

K. Jablon, MD
Department of Pediatrics, UCSF Benioff Children's Hospital,
1975 4th St, San Francisco, CA 94158, USA
e-mail: kimberly.jablon@ucsf.edu

E. Mathes, MD (✉)
Departments of Dermatology and Pediatrics, University of California, San Francisco,
1701 Divisadero Street, Third Floor, San Francisco, CA 94115, USA
e-mail: erin.mathes@ucsf.edu

© Springer International Publishing Switzerland 2016   131
M. Hogeling (ed.), *Case-Based Inpatient Pediatric Dermatology*,
DOI 10.1007/978-3-319-31569-0_8

Case 8.1

History

A 1-week-old term baby girl born to a 35-year-old G1P1 mom presents with ery-thematous nodules over her trunk, arms, buttocks, and thighs, which developed within the first week of life. She was born via forceps-assisted vaginal delivery for non-reassuring fetal heart tracing after 14 h of labor. Apgar scores were 1 and 7 at 1 and 5 min of life, respectively. She was floppy and cyanotic at birth. She recovered and cried spontaneously after 30 s of positive pressure ventilation. Her mother has a history of gestational diabetes and deep vein thrombosis 5 years ago, which was treated with enoxaparin during pregnancy. The nodules seem painful at times. Parents have given her Tylenol with unclear relief. She also has been sleepier in the past few days with some hard stools.

Physical Exam (Fig. 8.1)

Exam reveals an afebrile, well-nourished sleepy infant with multiple erythematous nodules on her extensor arms, back, buttocks, and thighs. Some of the nodules are fluctuant centrally.

Laboratory Parameters

- Platelet count: $145 \times 10^3 \ \mu L^{-1}$ ($150–450 \times 10^3 \ \mu L^{-1}$)
- White blood cell count: $12,000 \times 10^3$ cells/μL ($5240–9740$ cells/μL)
- Eosinophils: 5 %
- Calcium: 12 mg/dL (8.5–10.2 mg/dL)
- Creatinine 0.79 mg/dL (0–0.7 mg/dL)

Questions

1. What are the risk factors and epidemiology of this condition?
2. What monitoring and treatment would you consider?

Fig. 8.1 Subcutaneous fat
necrosis of the newborn

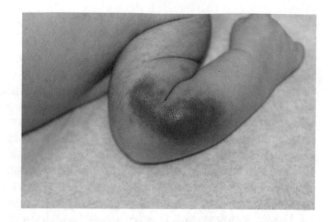

Answer

Subcutaneous fat necrosis of the newborn (SCFN) is a rare disorder that presents with focal or diffuse nodules within the first few weeks of life. The nodules usually completely resolve on their own over a few months with no residual skin changes, although there may be subcutaneous atrophy. While the prognosis is good, the range in severity can be quite broad, and complications like hypercalcemia, thrombocytopenia, and dyslipidemia can be seen. Rarely, hypercalcemia may be serious and can cause cardiac arrhythmia, coma, and even death. The most common areas involved are the trunk, arms, head and cervical areas, and legs.

The pathophysiology of subcutaneous fat necrosis is not entirely clear. The pathogenesis likely involves hypoxemia, cutaneous trauma, or stress, as suggested by the risk factors present in many cases. Newborns often have general poor condition around the time of birth including higher rates of infection. Specific risk factors around delivery include the use of forceps, hypoxic ischemic events, or hypothermia [1]. Patients who are treated with therapeutic cooling for hypoxic ischemic encephalopathy are particularly at risk [2]. Maternal risk factors include gestational diabetes mellitus and high blood pressure. Some patients also have risk factors for increased thrombosis such as family history of unexplained deep vein thrombosis, anti-phospholipid syndrome, or dyslipidemia which may point to another element of pathogenesis that has not been as well described [1]. There is no effect of gender or race, and patients are usually born at term.

The diagnosis is usually clear given the specific age of presentation and exam findings, but the differential may include cellulitis and soft tissue infection if localized. SCFN can be diagnosed clinically, although if the diagnosis is unclear, skin biopsy can be performed and reveals granulomatous necrosis in the subcutis with crystal like structures in the adipocytes.

Monitoring and Treatment

Serum calcium levels should be monitored in newborns with subcutaneous fat necrosis based on the severity of presentation, as there are no formal recommendations. Hypercalcemia has been detected a few months after diagnosis, which supports longer term monitoring. Newborns with singular lesions may be monitored clinically by their pediatricians, whereas newborns with severe presentations should have serum calcium checked up to every 2–4 weeks until age 4–6 months. The exact cause of hypercalcemia is unknown, but may be due to increased intestinal absorption due to macrophage release of 1,25-dihydroxyvitamin D3, or osteoclast activation from increased prostaglandin activity [3]. Other reported lab derangements include hypoglycemia, thrombocytopenia, hypertriglyceridemia, and eosinophilia [3, 4]. Mild hypercalcemia may be managed with a low calcium and vitamin D diet, such as withholding vitamin D supplementation for newborns with active disease. For severe cases, IV hydration and systemic treatment may be necessary. Furosemide, prednisone, and pamidronate are the most commonly used medications for treatment. Calcium deposits in kidneys, vessels, and other organs have been reported; however, there do not seem to be clinical complications from these deposits [1, 4].

In addition to the laboratory studies above, for this patient we would consider admission for hydration and monitoring. Given the elevated calcium, ionized calcium should be checked now and with future lab draws. Calcium should be checked weekly at first and then monthly until 4–6 months of age once it normalizes.

Case 8.2. Aplasia Cutis Congenita

History

A newborn male infant born to a 28-year-old G1P1 mom presents with a large stellate ulceration on his scalp. He is otherwise healthy with Apgar scores of 9 and 9 at 1 and 5 min of life. The infant's mother did not take any medications during pregnancy. There was no family history of skin disorders or genetic abnormalities.

Physical Exam (Fig. 8.2)

Exam reveals a non-dysmorphic infant in no acute distress with normal vital signs and growth parameters. On the midline scalp there is a 5 cm long and 1.5 cm wide ulceration with hemorrhagic crust. To the right of the central ulceration there is another 1.5 by 1.5 cm ulceration with hemorrhagic crust. Anterior and to the left there are erythematous, alopecic, and atrophic patches. There is relative alopecia extending from the frontal scalp to the vertex. There is no skin fragility on the body

Fig. 8.2 Aplasia cutis
(photograph courtesy of
Marcia Hogeling, M.D.)

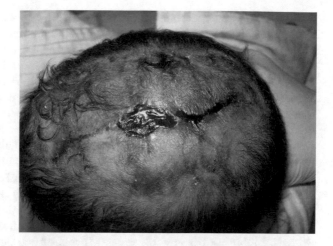

and no other birthmarks are present. Teeth and nails are normal. The neurological
exam is normal.

Imaging

- X-ray of the skull: non-ossification of the portion correlating to the skin lesion.
- MRI of the brain showed normal anatomy and development, without sagittal
  sinus thrombosis.

Questions

1. What other abnormalities can be associated with aplasia cutis congenita?
2. What diagnostic investigations should be performed?
3. What are the management options?

Answer

Aplasia cutis congenita (ACC) is a rare heterogeneous condition of localized or
widespread absence of skin at birth. The size of ACC lesions can vary widely from
small superficial lesions, to large defects on the scalp or body. Children can be born
with atrophic scars if lesions form early in gestation and heal in utero. The cause of
disruption in skin development varies and may include genetic abnormalities,
embryologic factors, teratogens, vascular disruption, or trauma [5–7].

ACC can occur in isolation or as part of other malformations and genetic syndromes. The most common form is isolated membranous aplasia cutis, usually found on the scalp and thought to be caused by incomplete closure of embryonic fusion lines [7]. It is most commonly sporadic, but can be inherited, usually in an autosomal dominant pattern [6]. Scalp ACC may also be found in association with limb abnormalities, such as limb reduction, skin tags, cutis marmorata, or nail dystrophy. Others have described scalp lesions together with epidermal and organoid nevi, which are usually caused by sporadic mutations, and may be associated with neurologic or ophthalmologic findings. ACC of the extremities (also called congenital localized absence of skin) has been reported in isolation and in association with epidermolysis bullosa (EB). In the setting of EB, ACC is associated with blistering and skin fragility [6]. Teratogens such as varicella, herpes simplex, methimazole, and alcohol can lead to ACC [6, 8]. Finally, ACC has been reported in many other genetic syndromes, including trisomy 13, several forms of ectodermal dysplasia, and 4p deletion syndrome [6].

Monitoring and Treatment

The diverse group of conditions associated with ACC emphasizes the importance of a full medical evaluation, focusing on areas such as the central nervous system, other ectodermal structures, and extremities, to ensure no other abnormalities are present [6, 8]. Isolated membranous aplasia cutis on the scalp usually requires no further investigation. However, some lesions may be associated with underlying CNS defects or sinus connections. Although imaging guidelines for ACC are controversial, most dermatologists agree an MRI of the brain should be obtained for larger lesions with underlying bony defects, lesions with palpable nodules, midline lesions between the vertex and occiput, and lesions associated with hypertrichosis, vascular lesions, or dimples [7]. Referral to a pediatric dermatologist is recommended in all cases of ACC to determine what additional workup is warranted.

Management depends on the extent of the lesion and associated complications. In the majority of cases with ulceration, simple wound care with daily cleansing and application of a petroleum-based ointment is appropriate [6, 9]. Even small defects of underlying bone usually ossify without treatment. When lesions are greater than 3–4 cm, especially if there is an underlying bony defect, grafting is often recommended, as larger lesions are more often associated with hemorrhage, venous thrombosis, and meningitis if located on the scalp. Death in cases of ACC can rarely occur from sagittal sinus hemorrhage, usually caused by the dura tearing from the tension of an eschar. As mentioned above, imaging of large lesions should occur before surgical intervention, as lesions associated with intracranial vascular abnormalities or those that affect dura or galea confer higher risk of surgical complications [7, 9].

For this patient, in addition to the skull X-ray and brain MRI, we would recommend a careful physical examination and medical history, and consider neurology and genetics consults to look for any subtle dysmorphic features. Wound care should be petrolatum to open areas, covered with Vaseline gauze, and a non-adherent dressing. The dressings can be held in place with Flexinet, or a hat. Monitoring for adequate healing and wound infection should occur frequently. This ulceration will take at least several weeks to heal.

Case 8.3. Giant Congenital Melanocytic Nevus

History

A newborn male presents with a large dark brown lesion extending over most of his back, buttocks, and thighs with the greatest diameter measuring greater than 20 cm. He was born at term without complications to a 28-year-old G1P1 mother with an uneventful prenatal course. There is no family history of congenital nevi or melanoma.

Physical Exam (Fig. 8.3)

Physical exam reveals a well-appearing infant in no distress with a large heterogeneous brown plaque covering most of the back, buttocks, and upper thighs. There are multiple dark brown and brown-pink plaques within, and mild hypertrichosis of the superior portion. There are approximately 20 0.5–2 cm uniformly pigmented light brown papules and plaques that are scattered on the arms, legs, trunk, and face, discontiguous with the main nevus. There is a small ulceration in the gluteal cleft.

Imaging

MRI of the brain and spine reveals no evidence of neurocutaneous melanosis (NCM), or hydrocephalus. There is no evidence of tethered cord or spinal dysraphism.

Questions

1. What are the risks associated with congenital melanocytic nevi?
2. What diagnostic investigations should be performed?
3. What are the treatment options?

Fig. 8.3 Large congenital
melanocytic nevus
(photograph courtesy of
Marcia Hogeling, M.D.)

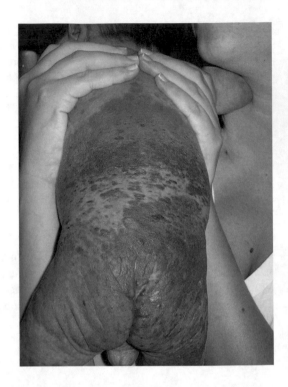

Answer

Congenital melanocytic nevi (CMN) are abnormal collections of melanocytes in ectopic locations that are present at birth, or develop in the first few weeks of life. While a new classification system has been proposed, most commonly CMN are classified as small if less than 1.5 cm, medium if between 1.5 and 19.9 cm, or giant if measuring greater than 20 cm by adulthood [10]. CMN tend to grow proportionately to the growth of the child, and a nomogram can be used to predict adult size [10]. CMN are common, occurring in about 1 % of all newborns, with higher rates in girls than boys [11]. Fortunately, giant CMN are rare, occurring in approximately 1 in 20,000 newborns [11, 12]. They present as hyperpigmented macules, patches, and plaques, most commonly on the trunk, followed by the extremities, head, and neck. They can have varying degrees of color variation, hypertrichosis, nodularity, or ulceration. In large CMN, satellite lesions (smaller nevi that are discontiguous with the main nevus) can be present and can increase in number throughout life. The differential diagnosis includes other nevi such as epidermal nevus, nevus sebaceous, plexiform neurofibromas, café au lait macules, and dermal melanocytosis.

The major medical risks of CMN include the development of NCM, and malignant melanoma. NCM is a rare syndrome in which patients have melanocyte deposition in the central nervous system in association with either a giant CMN, or three or more smaller CMN. Risk factors include multiple satellite lesions (especially greater than 20), and perhaps location on the posterior axis [13, 14]. Patients may be asymptomatic, or present with seizures, hydrocephalus, or developmental delay [12, 15]. The majority of patients present under 2 years of age, and almost all before age 5 [10]. Prognosis varies, although death from neurologic complications is not uncommon, ranging from 8 to 21 % [10]. All patients with neurologic findings, as well as patients with a large CMN with >20 satellite lesions, or three or more inter-mediate CMNs should have a screening MRI of the brain and spine before 6 months of age, as there may be neurosurgical interventions that could alleviate symptoms [16]. Approximately 1/3 of patients with melanosis on imaging are asymptomatic [10]. These patients should be followed by a pediatric neurologist and with repeat imaging as clinically indicated [12, 16].

The rate at which CMN can give rise to malignant melanoma varies in the litera-ture, due to differences in follow-up times, inclusion of benign proliferative nodules, and distinctions between extra-cutaneous and cutaneous melanoma [10]. It is esti-mated that the overall risk of cutaneous melanoma is about 0.7 % for all CMN [13], although the risk of malignancy correlates with greater size of the lesion. The life-time risk of malignancy is reported as less than 1 % in small and medium sized CMN [14], while reports for giant CMN range from 2.5 to 6.3 % [13, 17]. A significant number of cutaneous melanomas in larger CMN are diagnosed under age 5 [14, 15, 18]. It is not known whether truncal location is a risk factor independent of CMN size. While satellite nevi are associated with NCM, they have not shown to increase risk for cutaneous melanoma. Malignant melanoma can present in the CMN itself, or the first symptoms may be of non-cutaneous melanoma in the CNS, or gut mucosa.

Management depends on the size of the lesion, location, and experience of the surgeon. Treatment goals include decreasing risk of malignant melanoma, and improving aesthetics and psychosocial well-being. It is acceptable to monitor CMN without intervention in all cases, and especially if excision would cause loss of function and in cases of symptomatic NCM or CNS melanoma. The most accepted treatments are surgical modalities, which include serial excision, tissue expansion, and skin grafting. Serial excision has the best risk profile, but is limited to lesions that can be excised in 2–3 stages. Expansion and grafting can provide excellent outcomes, but with higher risk of surgical complications like infection or ischemia [12]. Nonsurgical treatments such as dermabrasion, laser, or chemical peels may decrease the nevus cell burden, but they do not result in complete cell removal, and can create challenges in monitoring for malignant changes posttreatment [11]. It is unclear whether surgical treatment of CMN decreases the risk of melanoma, but it is important to remember that complete removal of all of the melanocytes in a giant CMN is virtually impossible, and melanomas can present deep to the excised areas.

For this patient, in addition to the baseline MRI of the brain and spine, we would recommend periodic examination by a pediatric dermatologist. If the parents are interested in serial excision of the more visible parts of the nevus, they should be referred to an experienced plastic surgeon. If firm areas, nodules, or other concern-ing features develop in the lesion, they should be biopsied for histologic evaluation. Referral to patient support groups such as Nevus Outreach can be very helpful for family and child adjustment.

Case 8.4. Neonatal Lupus

History

A term newborn male infant born to a 36-year-old G1P1 mom is noted to have cutaneous lesions on her face and scalp in the newborn nursery. He is otherwise healthy and the delivery was uncomplicated. His mother had no prenatal complications and has no medical problems, aside from complaints of dry mouth. There is a family history of rheumatoid arthritis in the maternal grandmother, and no other autoimmune disorders. His mother was not taking any medications.

Physical Exam (Fig. 8.4)

The infant is well appearing with erythematous to violaceous plaques, some with central hypopigmentation and peripheral hyperpigmentation on the face, accentuated around the eyes. Cardiac and abdominal exam are normal.

Laboratory Parameters

- Platelet count: $70,000 \times 10^3 \, \mu L^{-1}$ ($150,000–450,000 \times 10^3 \, \mu L^{-1}$)
- Hemoglobin: 15 g/dL (13.5–17.5 g/dL)
- EKG: normal sinus rhythm

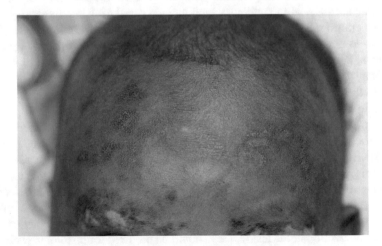

Fig. 8.4 Neonatal lupus

- Anti Ro antibody IgG positive
- Mother Anti-Ro Ab IgG positive
- AST 223 IU/L (10–40 IU/L), ALT 279 IU/L (7–56 IU/L), total bilirubin 4.7 mg/dL (0.3–1.2 mg/dL), GGT 278 IU/L (0–30 IU/L), Alk Phos 286 IU/L (35–125 IU/L)

Questions

1. What is the range of cutaneous findings in this condition?
2. What are the non-cutaneous findings of this disease and what screenings should be offered?
3. What are the treatments for this condition?

Answer

Neonatal lupus erythematosus (NLE) is a passively acquired autoimmune disease associated with maternal autoantibodies that are transmitted across the placenta, most commonly Anti Ro/SSA or Anti L/SSB. The major manifestations include cutaneous lesions and congenital heart block (CHB). Most cases with cutaneous manifestations present 2–4 weeks after birth, although some newborns may be born with cutaneous lesions. The cutaneous manifestations and other systemic findings usually resolve in 6 months when maternal antibodies are no longer present in infants, although the cardiac manifestations may last for years [19–21]. The incidence of cutaneous symptoms in newborns born to mothers with known SSA or SSB antibody is reported up to 20 %, with rates of complete CHB 1–2 % [22, 23]. More than half of mothers of children with NLE are reported to be asymptomatic prior to pregnancy; therefore, the suspicion for NLE should remain in patients with characteristic lesions, even if there is no maternal history of autoimmune disorders [20].

Cutaneous lesions are found in 50–70 % of all newborns with NLE and usually present as annular erythematous plaques or patches with fine scale, or rarely thick crusts. Unlike discoid lupus, there is usually no residual atrophy or scarring once healed. Another common manifestation is the distinctive periorbital "owl eye" or "eye mask" facial rash, which if present can point the examiner towards NLE. Most newborns exhibit annular erythematous lesions in sun-exposed areas such as the face and scalp, followed by arms and legs, and lastly trunk and groin. Other less common cutaneous findings include petechiae, persistent cutis marmorata, discoid lesions, or congenital atrophic scarring. The diagnosis of neonatal lupus is often under-recognized, and lesions are misdiagnosed as tinea corporis or eczema. The natural course is complete resolution over 6–7 months with no residual skin changes, mild telangiectasia, or dyspigmentation [21].

NLE cases involving the heart are often the most severe, with mortality for CHB reported up to 16% [19]. Dilated cardiomyopathy is another reported cardiac finding associated with NLE, as are various anatomic lesions which may be unrelated to CHB [19]. Neonates with CHB may require long-term pacing with a pacemaker in up to two-thirds of cases [19, 20]. Early screening and detection in gestation can be helpful in preventing complications, especially if the mom has known antibodies or previous children with NLE. While there are no formal guidelines, these mothers are often monitored frequently with fetal echocardiography after the first trimester. However, there are still cases of fetal mortality from hydrops. Although the skin and heart are the main organs affected in NLE, extracutaneous manifestations also include hematologic or hepatobiliary findings. Hematologic findings include thrombocytopenia and anemia, while liver disease manifests most commonly as transaminitis or hepatic cholestasis [20, 21]. Like the cutaneous lesions, hematologic and hepatic findings self-resolve at approximately 6 months of age [20, 21]. Rarely, kidney and central nervous system involvement have been reported, although newborns are not routinely screened for these manifestations [20].

Low-to-mid potency topical steroids and sun protection are the mainstays of treatment for cutaneous lesions [23]. Intravenous steroids or IVIG can be used for more severe hepatobiliary or hematologic findings. Pacemakers may be implanted for children who do not recover from CHB. In the long term, both mothers and patients should be monitored for the development of autoimmune disease [20, 21].

For this patient with cutaneous findings suggesting neonatal lupus, and no preexisting diagnosis of CHB, we would recommend an electrocardiogram, liver function tests, a CBC, serum creatinine, and urinalysis. In addition, both baby and mother should be screened for antinuclear, anti-double stranded DNA, anti-SSA/Ro, anti-SSB/La, and anti-U1-RNP antibodies. This child's thrombocytopenia and hepatitis should be closely followed and treated if necessary, usually with systemic corticosteroids. Low potency topical steroids and sun protection should be used to treat and prevent the cutaneous lesions. Pediatric rheumatology and dermatology should be involved in the care of a patient with NLE and systemic findings.

Case 8.5. Incontinentia Pigmenti

History

A 4-day-old female infant born at term presents with linear vesicles and bullae developing on her extremities. She was born to a 28-year-old G3P1 with history of two spontaneous abortions and oligohydramnios in pregnancy. She is otherwise healthy with no fevers or other vital sign abnormalities, and adequate weight gain. She is being treated with IV acyclovir for presumed HSV, but the lesions are not improving.

Fig. 8.5 Incontinentia pigmenti

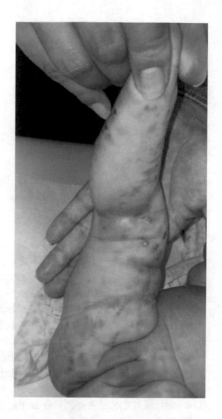

Physical Exam (Fig. 8.5)

Well-appearing infant in no acute distress with hyperpigmented, erythematous and crusted plaques, papules and vesicles in a blashkolinear array on her right posterior leg, thigh, buttock, and vulva. She also has two 1 cm crusted plaques on her vertex and occipital scalp. Neurologic exam is normal.

Laboratory Parameters

- Eosinophils 4.61×10^9 L^{-1} ($0–1.0 \times 10^9$ L^{-1})
- WBC 15×10^9 L^{-1} ($6–14 \times 10^9$ L^{-1})
- Skin HSV PCR negative
- Bacterial culture of skin and blood—no growth

Histopathology

Intraepidermal spongiosis with eosinophilic and neutrophilic infiltration. Keratinocytes are large and dyskeratotic.

Questions

1. What are the stages of cutaneous changes in incontinentia pigmenti?
2. What additional workup should be performed?

Answers

Incontinentia pigmenti (IP) is a rare X-linked dominant disorder that universally affects the skin and can also affect other ectodermal tissues such as teeth, eyes, central nervous system, and skeletal system. It is usually lethal to males; therefore the vast majority of babies with IP are females. The skin manifestations are characterized by mosaicism, an expression of two or more different cell lines [24]. Expression of IP is variable, as the majority of women have non-random X chromosome inactivation, with the mutation selected against around the time of birth [24]. The mutation that causes IP is in the gene IKBKG or NEMO, which codes for the transcription factor NF-kappa B essential modulator, a protein involved in the immune system, inflammation, and apoptosis [24, 25].

The skin lesions in IP are in a linear pattern and evolve through four stages, some of which may overlap or not develop at all. They begin as vesicles or bullae on an erythematous base in the neonate, following the lines of Blaschko. The lesions evolve into hyperkeratotic verrucous plaques at a few months of life. This is followed by hyperpigmentation which may or may not correspond to areas of prior lesions, and lasts until about 16 months [24]. Finally, hypopigmentation or depigmented lesions are seen in adulthood, along with atrophy and absence of hair and sweat glands [25], most commonly on the lower extremities [24]. The initial lesions have eosinophils, which are thought to be an inflammatory response to the cells with a defective X chromosome [24], and may be associated with peripheral eosinophilia or leukocytosis [25]. Nails can be affected with findings varying from fragile nails, to yellowish pigmentation, hyperkeratosis, and onycholysis [24]. The cutaneous lesions of IP should be treated with simple wound care while in the vesicular and crusted stage.

If IP is suspected in the newborn, an urgent ophthalmologic exam and neurologic workup are warranted. A dental exam should be performed once teeth start to erupt. Dental anomalies associated with IP include hypodontia, delayed eruption of teeth, conical teeth, or partial anodontia (lack of teeth) [24]. Ophthalmic anomalies such as retinal vasculopathy, strabismus, or cataracts are the most common extracutaneous findings, occurring in 35–77 % of patients [25]. Retinal vasculopathy can lead to detachment, bleeding fibrosis, and rarely blindness [25], thus urgent consultation is necessary. Central nervous system findings occur in 10–30 %, and may include seizures, mental retardation, ataxia, spastic abnormalities, cerebral atrophy, hypoplasia of the corpus callosum, encephalitis, ischemic strokes, and hydrocephalus [24]. Other disorders with similar lesions in newborns should be eliminated as part of the workup, including neonatal herpes, congenital neonatal bullous disorders, or impetigo [26]. Later lesions of IP can be confused with epidermal nevi, pigmentary mosaicism, and other blashkolinear birthmarks. Skin biopsy can usually distinguish amongst these conditions.

Genetic testing for mutations in IKBKG is commercially available and can be used to confirm the diagnosis and assess carrier state of unaffected females. Approximately 80 % of patients with IP will have a mutation in IKBKG [27].

In addition to a skin biopsy to confirm the diagnosis, this infant should be referred for an urgent ophthalmologic exam and to see genetics and neurology. Genetic testing can be pursued especially for counseling for future family planning. Crusted areas can be covered with petrolatum to speed healing.

References

1. Mahé E, Girszyn N, Hadj-Rabia S, et al. Subcutaneous fat necrosis of the newborn: a systematic evaluation of risk factors, clinical manifestations, complications and outcome of 16 children. Br J Dermatol. 2007;156:709–15.
2. Grass B, Weibel L, Hagmann C, et al. Subcutaneous fat necrosis in neonates with hypoxic ischaemic encephalopathy registered in the Swiss National Asphyxia and Cooling Register. BMC Pediatr. 2015;15:73.
3. Samedi V, Yusuf K, Yee W, et al. Neonatal hypercalcemia secondary to subcutaneous fat necrosis successfully treated with pamidronate: a case series and literature review. Am J Perinatol. 2014;4(2):93–6.
4. Shumer D, Thaker V, Taylor G, et al. Severe hypercalcaemia due to subcutaneous fat necrosis: presentation, management and complications. Arch Dis Child Fetal Neonatal Ed. 2014;99:419–21.
5. Brzezinski P, Pinteala AE, Foia L, et al. Aplasia cutis congenita of the scalp—what are the steps to be followed? Case report and review of the literature. An Bras Dermatol. 2015;90(1):100–3.
6. Frieden IJ. Aplasia cutis congenita: a clinical review and proposal for classification. J Am Acad Dermatol. 1986;14:646–60.
7. Eichenfield LF, Frieden IJ, Mathes EF, Zaenglein AL, editors. Neonatal and infant dermatology. 3rd ed. Philadelphia: Elsevier Saunders; 2015.
8. Evers ME, Steijlen PM, Hamel BC. Aplasia cutis congenita and associated disorders: an update. Clin Genet. 1995;47(6):295–301.
9. Burkhead JA, Poindexter G, Morrell DS. A case of extensive aplasia cutis congenita with underlying skull defect and central nervous system malformation: discussion of large skin defects, complications, treatment and outcome. J Perinatol. 2009;29:582–4.
10. Krengel S, Scope A, Dusza SW, Vonthein R, Marghoob AA. New recommendations for the categorization of cutaneous features of congenital melanocytic nevi. J Am Acad Dermatol. 2013;68(3):441–51.

11. Arneja JS, Gosain AK. Giant congenital melanocytic nevi. Plast Reconstr Surg. 2007;120(2):26–40.
12. Marano AA, Feintisch AM, Datiashvili R. Giant congenital melanocytic nevus of the buttock. Eplasty. 2015;5:31.
13. Krengel S, Marghoob AA. Current management approaches for congenital melanocytic nevi. Dermatol Clin. 2012;30(3):377–87.
14. Price HN, Schaffer JV. Congenital melanocytic nevi-when to worry and how to treat: facts and controversies. Clin Dermatol. 2010;28(3):293–302.
15. Araujo C, Resende C, Pardal F, et al. Giant congenital melanocytic nevi and neurocutaneous melanosis. Case Rep Med. 2015;2015:545603.
16. Frieden IJ, Williams ML, Barkovich AJ. Giant congenital melanocytic nevi: brain magnetic resonance findings in neurologically asymptomatic children. J Am Acad Dermatol. 1994;31(3):423–9.
17. Rhodes AR, Wood WC, Sober AJ, Mihm Jr MC. Nonepidermal origin of malignant melanoma associated with a giant congenital nevocellular nevus. Plast Reconstr Surg. 1981;67(6):782–90.
18. Bittencourt FV, Marghoob AA, Kopf AW, et al. Large congenital melanocytic nevi and the risk for development of malignant melanoma and neurocutaneous melanocytosis. Pediatrics. 2000;106(4):736–41.
19. Eronen M, Siren M, Ekblad H, et al. Short- and long-term outcome of children with congenital complete heart block diagnosed in utero or as a newborn. Pediatrics. 2000;106(1):86–91.
20. Li YQ, Wang Q, Luo Y, et al. Neonatal lupus erythematosus: a review of 123 cases in China. Int J Rheum Dis. 2015;18(7):761–7.
21. Weston WL, Morelli JG, Lee LA. The clinical spectrum of anti-Ro-positive cutaneous neonatal lupus erythematosus. J Am Acad Dermatol. 1999;40(5 Pt 1):675–81.
22. Cimaz R, Spence DL, Hornberger L, Silverman ED. Incidence and spectrum of neonatal lupus erythematosus: a prospective study of infants born to mothers with anti-Ro autoantibodies. J Pediatr. 2003;142(6):678–83.
23. Hasbún T, Chamlin SL. A 6-week-old boy with annular skin lesions. Neonatal lupus erythematosus. Pediatr Ann. 2014;43(1):1–3.
24. Poziomczyk CS, Recuero JK, Bringhenti L. Incontinentia pigmenti. An Bras Dermatol. 2014;89(1):26–36.
25. Ehrenreich M, Tarlow MM, Godlewska-Janusz E, Schwartz RA. Incontinentia pigmenti (Bloch-Sulzberger syndrome): a systemic disorder. Cutis. 2007;79(5):355–62.
26. Yang Y, Guo Y, Ping Y, et al. Neonatal incontinentia pigmenti: six cases and a literature review. Exp Ther Med. 2014;8(6):1797–806.
27. Aradhya S, Woffendin H, Jakins T, et al. A recurrent deletion in the ubiquitously expressed NEMO (IKK-gamma) gene accounts for the vast majority of incontinentia pigmenti mutations. Hum Mol Genet. 2001;10:2171–9.

Chapter 9
Neoplastic and Infiltrative Diseases

Ellen S. Haddock and Wynnis L. Tom

Abstract Several pediatric neoplasms present as nonspecific pink, red-blue, or purple-colored nodules on the skin. A benign process versus one of malignant potential can be difficult to determine clinically, making index of suspicion and histologic examination important. This chapter highlights four neoplastic conditions that may present in early childhood and uses a case-based approach to discuss the appropriate workup.

Keywords Neoplastic • Cancer • Leukemia cutis • Acute lymphoid leukemia • Acute myeloid leukemia • Blueberry muffin phenotype • Neuroblastoma • Fibrosarcoma • Infantile myofibroma • Myofibromatosis

Abbreviations

ALL	Acute lymphoid leukemia
AML	Acute myeloid leukemia
BCL	B cell lymphoma
CBC	Complete blood count
CT	Computed tomography
FISH	Fluorescence in situ hybridization
GLUT1	Glucose transporter 1
HVA	Homovanillic acid
LDH	Lactate dehydrogenase
MIBG	Metaiodobenzylguanidine

E.S. Haddock, MBA
School of Medicine, University of California, San Diego and Pediatric & Adolescent Dermatology, Rady Children's Hospital, 8010 Frost Street, Suite 602, San Diego, CA 92123, USA
e-mail: ehaddock@ucsd.edu

W.L. Tom, MD (✉)
Departments of Dermatology and Pediatrics, University of California, San Diego and Rady Children's Hospital, 8010 Frost Street, Suite 602, San Diego, CA 92123, USA
e-mail: wtom@rchsd.org

© Springer International Publishing Switzerland 2016   147
M. Hogeling (ed.), *Case-Based Inpatient Pediatric Dermatology*,
DOI 10.1007/978-3-319-31569-0_9

MLL	Mixed lineage leukemia
MRI	Magnetic resonance imaging
NB84	Neuroblastoma 84
NFP	Neurofilament protein
NSE	Neuron-specific enolase
NTRK3	Neurotrophic tyrosine kinase receptor type 3
Pax-5	Paired box 5
PCR	Polymerase chain reaction
PELVIS	Perineal hemangioma, external genitalia malformations, lipomyelo-meningocele, vesicorenal abnormalities, imperforate anus, skin tag
PGP9.5	Protein gene product 9.5
PHOX2B	Paired-like homeobox 2b
SMA	Smooth muscle actin
TdT	Terminal deoxynucleotidyl transferase
TORCH	Toxoplasmosis, other, rubella, cytomegalovirus, herpes
TSEB	Total skin electron beam
VMA	Vanillylmandelic acid

Case 9.1

History

A baby girl is born at 38 weeks by C-section due to intolerance of labor after an uneventful pregnancy. Her APGAR (Appearance, Pulse, Grimace, Activity, Respiration) scores at 1 and 5 min were 1 and 3, respectively. She is observed to have scattered purplish lesions diffusely on the skin (Figs. 9.1 and 9.2).

Physical Exam

On physical exam, she has 20 erythematous to violaceous macules, plaques, and firm nodules over her face, neck, and trunk. The lesions are unchanged with rubbing; they do not blanch or become more swollen (negative Darier's sign).

Questions

1. What is your differential diagnosis?
2. What are the next steps?

Fig. 9.1 Multiple
violaceous nodules on the
face of a newborn girl.
With permission © 2015
[Alvin Coda, M.D.]

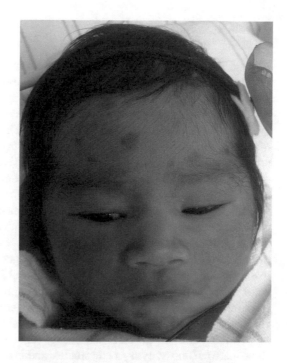

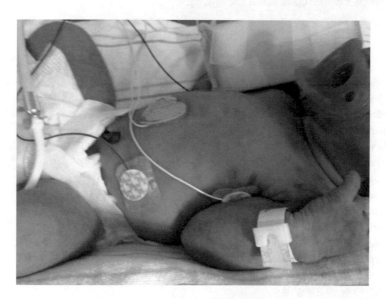

Fig. 9.2 Similar lesions scattered on the trunk. With permission © 2015 [Sheila Friedlander, M.D.]

Answers

This newborn baby with scattered erythematous to violaceous skin lesions has a "blueberry muffin" phenotype. This may be caused by dermal erythropoiesis due to congenital infections, including toxoplasmosis, syphilis, rubella, and cytomegalovirus (TORCH infections); hemolytic disease of the newborn and hereditary spherocytosis; and twin–twin perfusion syndrome. The phenotype can also be due to neoplastic infiltrative processes such as rhabdomyosarcoma, metastatic neuroblastoma, leukemia cutis, and malignant histiocytosis [1, 2]. Leukemoid proliferations such as the transient myeloproliferative disorder associated with trisomy 21 or exogenous stressors are additional causes [3, 4].

An infant with blueberry muffin phenotype must be worked up for these multiple potential etiologies. A white blood cell count with differential and peripheral smear can help distinguish congenital leukemia cutis from a leukemoid reaction, as an orderly left shift with white blood cells in all stages of maturation would be expected in a leukemoid reaction, while in leukemia cutis, blast cells and mature forms would be expected to dominate with fewer cells in the middle stages of development [4]. Initial workup should also include enzyme-linked immunosorbent assay to test for antibodies to congenital infections, Coomb's test for hemolytic disease of the newborn, urinary and serum catecholamines to rule out neuroblastoma, and skin biopsy. Bone marrow biopsy, cytogenetic studies, and imaging to rule out other extramedullary lesions may be considered later [4, 5].

Lab Results

- White blood count: 7.7 (normal range 9–29 thousand/μL)
- Absolute neutrophil count: 3760 (6000–23,500 μL)
- Hemoglobin: 12.1 (14–22 g/dL)
- Hematocrit: 36.1 (42–64%)
- MCV: 105.4 (102–115 fL)
- Platelets: 224 (140–440 TH/μL)
- C-reactive protein: <0.5 (0–0.99 mg/dL)
- Total bilirubin: 5.9 (1.1–11.3 mg/dL)
- Lactate dehydrogenase (LDH): 7042 (934–2150 U/L)
- Uric acid: 7.7 (1.9–7.9 mg/dL)
- Urine homovanillic acid (HVA): 27.6 (9.1–36 mg/g creat)
- Urine vanillylmandelic acid (VMA): <10.5 (5.5–26 mg/g creat)
- Blood: type O positive (same as mother's)
- IgM: <5 (1–57 mg/dL)

Peripheral Smear

The absolute neutrophil count is decreased at 3760. Red cells are normal in number and morphology. The white cell count is mildly decreased and notable for hypersegmentation of eosinophils, relative monocytopenia, and mild absolute neutropenia. No definitive blast population is identified. Platelets are normal in number, with scattered large platelets seen.

Abdominal Ultrasound

No intra-abdominal or retroperitoneal mass. Adrenal glands are normal.

Punch Biopsy from Left Leg Lesion

There are sheets of atypical cells infiltrating the dermis and subcutaneous fat. The atypical cells have high nuclear-to-cytoplasm ratios, hyperchromatic nuclei, irregular nuclear borders, and scant to moderate amounts of amphophilic cytoplasm. Abundant karyorrhectic debris is seen. The mitotic rate is high. There is no evidence of necrosis. The neoplastic cells infiltrate surrounding adnexal structures and separate collagen bundles.

- Synaptophysin: neoplastic cells negative.
- CD3: neoplastic cells negative.
- CD20: neoplastic cells negative.
- CD45: neoplastic cells diffusely positive.
- CD79a (integrated): neoplastic cells negative.
- CD99: neoplastic cells negative.
- Myogenin: neoplastic cells negative.
- Ki-67: approximately 90 % nuclear positivity in neoplastic cells.
- Myeloperoxidase (integrated): neoplastic cells diffusely and strongly positive.
- BCL-2 (integrated): scattered cells positive.
- BCL-6 (integrated): neoplastic cells negative.
- TdT (integrated): neoplastic cells negative.

Flow Cytometry of Skin Cells

No immunophenotypic evidence of acute leukemia, high-grade myelodysplastic syndrome, or T-cell neoplasm. Minimal population (<1 %) of abnormal lymphocytes.

CSF

Rare atypical cells of uncertain significance in a background of peripheral blood. No cytoplasmic granules or Auer rods.

Bone Marrow Biopsy

Hypercellular marrow at approximately 98% cellularity. Megakaryocytes are increased in number and show a generally unremarkable morphology. Relative myeloid hypoplasia, with myeloid lineage cells showing hypogranulation and nuclear hypersegmentation. No cytoplasmic granules or Auer rods.

- Blasts: 5%
- Metamyelocytes/myelocytes: 8%
- Bands: 8%
- Neutrophils: 26%
- Lymphocytes: 21%
- Eosinophils: 6%
- Monocytes: 6.5%
- Erythroid precursors: 19.5%

Case Discussion

This infant's IgM screen was negative, ruling out TORCH infections, and since she had the same blood type as her mother and a normal bilirubin level, hemolytic disease of the newborn was unlikely. Normal VMA and HVA along with a normal abdominal ultrasound made neuroblastoma unlikely, but her high LDH was concerning for tumor lysis syndrome. Her skin biopsy showed neoplastic cells and immunostaining strongly positive for myeloperoxidase, consistent with cutaneous myelogenous leukemia. Although peripheral blood smear and bone marrow biopsy did not show a significantly elevated blast population, chromosomal analysis of marrow cells later confirmed that she had a t(11;19) translocation with involvement of the Mixed Lineage Leukemia (MLL) gene at 11q23, consistent with acute myelogenous leukemia.

Leukemia cutis is a cutaneous manifestation of leukemia, with infiltration of the skin and subcutaneous tissue by malignant myeloid or lymphoid blasts [3, 6, 7]. It is more common in males than females (2:1) [4]. Leukemia is the most common malignancy of childhood, and leukemia cutis occurs in 2–30% of patients with acute myeloid leukemia (AML) and 1–3% of patients with acute lymphocytic leukemia (ALL) [6, 8–14]. While congenital leukemia, defined as leukemia presenting at birth or within the first month of life, is relatively rare (1–8.6/10⁶ live births, less than 1% of all childhood leukemia), leukemia cutis is relatively common within the small subset of patients with congenital leukemia (25–64% of patients) and is the first sign in half of cases [1, 3, 15].

Leukemia cutis has a wide range of presentations, but the most common include flesh-colored, red-brown, or violaceous papules, nodules, and plaques. Lesions occur most often on the legs, but the arms, back, chest, scalp, and face are also common [6, 16]. They may also develop at sites of previous skin trauma [8, 17]. In congenital leukemia, skin lesions are often accompanied by purpura, petechiae, and ecchymoses, creating the blueberry muffin appearance that was seen in this case [3, 8]. Patients may have hepatosplenomegaly, lethargy, pallor, anemia, failure to thrive, and irritability due to bone pain [1, 4, 6, 15]. White blood cell count is usually high.

The pathogenesis of leukemia cutis is not well understood. Congenital leukemia cutis could be an abnormal continuation of the dermal erythropoiesis that normally occurs during the first 5 months of gestation [1, 18]. Whether blasts originate in the skin or are colonized by leukemic blasts from bone marrow has not been established [7]. Leukemia cutis is usually seen in conjunction with systemic leukemia, but in <10 % of cases it may be an isolated finding without any detectable bone marrow or peripheral blood involvement, referred to as aleukemic leukemia cutis. It is possible that aleukemic leukemia cutis reflects metastasis of undetectable bone marrow disease [3].

Biopsy of leukemia cutis typically reveals a dense diffuse or nodular infiltrate of the dermis and subcutis with perivascular or periadnexal involvement [6, 17]. The epidermis is usually unaffected, with a Grenz zone between the epidermis and the leukemic infiltrate [4]. The leukemic blasts are typically medium to large in size with a high nuclear-to-cytoplasmic ratio, smooth chromatin, prominent nucleoli, and increased mitotic activity [1, 19]. Leukemia cutis may look histologically similar to lymphomas, blastic plasmacytoid dendritic cell neoplasms, mast cell sarcomas, and plasma cell neoplasms. Immunohistochemistry or cytogenetics are typically required for definitive diagnosis [3, 20].

There is no consensus about which immunohistochemical stains are most sensitive for identifying myeloid leukemia cutis, and there is significant variability in staining results [7]. Even in the context of systemic leukemia, the diagnosis of leukemia cutis can be challenging because there can be discordance between the immunophenotype of leukemic skin cells and bone marrow cells within the same individual [7, 19]. Most leukemia cutis stains positive for CD45; however, in young children, leukemia cutis may instead stain positive for CD43 [21]. Expression of myeloperoxidase, CD117, and cathepsin-B support a diagnosis of myeloid leukemia cutis, while expression of CD3, CD10, CD20, CD99, paired box 5 (Pax-5), terminal deoxynucleotidyl transferase (TdT), and CD179 support a diagnosis of lymphoblastic leukemia cutis [21].

Cytogenetic analysis can be especially helpful when skin markers differ from bone marrow markers and is helpful in prognostication [22]. Chromosomal abnormalities are particularly common in congenital leukemia, with the most common being rearrangement of the MLL gene at 11q23, as seen in this case [1, 5]. In a Dutch series, this translocation was identified in 30.6 % of congenital leukemia cases in which cytogenetics was performed [15].

In general, the prognosis for leukemia cutis is poor. Congenital leukemia cutis carries the same prognosis as congenital leukemia overall [4], with survival at 24 months being only 23 % in one study of 109 patients [15]. Survival is higher in AML than ALL (24 % versus 14 %) [15]. Rarely, temporary or permanent spontaneous remission may occur in congenital leukemia [18, 23]. However, the majority of aleukemic leukemia cutis cases progress to systemic involvement within the next 4 months, and there are no reported cases of spontaneous remission when the 11q23 translocation is present, conferring poor prognosis [1, 3].

The baby described in this case presented with blueberry muffin phenotype and skin biopsy consistent with congenital leukemia cutis but no clear bone marrow evidence of disease. By 6 days after birth, her LDH had normalized and her blueberry muffin phenotype was resolving, so she was discharged from the hospital. In light of the cutaneous improvement, lack of bone marrow evidence for leukemia, and possibility of spontaneous resolution of leukemia cutis in some instances, she was followed closely without treatment. The skin lesions resolved completely by the age of 3 weeks, and her complete blood count (CBC) normalized aside from mild, persistent anemia.

However, results from chromosomal analysis of bone marrow cells returned, showing translocation (11;19) in 22% of metaphases. Fluorescence in situ hybridization (FISH) showed involvement of the mixed lineage leukemia (MLL) oncogene at 11q23. At 4 months of age, the patient developed new reddish papules along her hairline, followed by progressive development of bluish papules on her scalp, chest, abdomen, and groin, as well as having gum bleeding. She was found to have leukocytosis (30.1 thousand/μL) with peripheral blasts (45%), anemia, thrombocytopenia, elevated uric acid (9.9), and elevated LDH (8195). She was admitted to the hospital, and bone marrow biopsy showed AML with 62.5% blasts, the 11q23 translocation, and tetrasomy 8 (known to be associated with leukemia cutis [6]). She was treated for tumor lysis syndrome and started on a chemotherapy regimen including cytarabine, daunorubicin, and etoposide. After receiving three rounds of chemotherapy, she had no evidence of residual disease. In light of her high-risk cytogenetics, she underwent stem cell transplant at the age of 8 months when matched cord blood became available. Her course has been complicated by recurrence of disease half a year after the stem cell transplant. She was found to have marrow, extramedullary, and CNS involvement, and she has been treated with aggressive chemotherapy and a second hematopoietic stem cell transplant, with no disease recurrence to date.

In general, if leukemia cutis occurs in the context of systemic leukemia, the underlying systemic disease should be treated with intensive chemotherapy [6]. Cytarabine and anthracyclines are most commonly used in AML [24]. There is no consensus on treatment for aleukemic leukemic cutis. A recent review by Handler et al. recommends that unless the MLL 11q23 translocation is identified, systemic therapy should be delayed until systemic leukemia is diagnosed [1]. However, if the MLL translocation is identified, chemotherapy should be initiated immediately. For patients with the MLL gene rearrangement, hematopoietic stem cell transplant may be advised in addition to chemotherapy, although this is controversial as it was not associated with improved survival in a study of 756 patients [24, 25]. When chemotherapy produces bone marrow remission without resolving the skin involvement, total skin electron beam (TSEB) therapy can be useful to eradicate the skin lesions, which could otherwise re-seed the bone marrow and cause relapse of systemic disease [26, 27]. Patients with leukemia cutis are predisposed to extramedullary relapses and should be followed long term with scheduled physical exams and routine blood draws [27].

Case 9.2

History

A 7-month-old female presents with two bumps, on her left plantar foot and right labia majora, which have been growing slowly for the past 4 months. They do not seem to be painful or otherwise symptomatic. They are never red, nor do they bleed or have exudate. She has no other medical problems.

Physical Exam

She has a 6 mm firm, skin-colored nodule on the left plantar foot, which transilluminates (Fig. 9.3). She also has a similar 8 mm nodule on the right labia majora (Fig. 9.4). A hard mass is palpated in the left lower quadrant of the abdominal cavity.

Questions

1. What is in your differential diagnosis?
2. What are your next steps?

Answers

The differential diagnosis for one or more firm cutaneous nodules in an infant includes myofibroma, hemangiopericytoma (now considered part of the spectrum of myofibromatosis), leiomyoma, neuroblastoma, and fibrosarcoma. Detection of

Fig. 9.3 Skin-colored, slowly growing nodule on the left plantar foot of a 7-month-old female. With permission © 2015 [Sheila Friedlander, M.D.]

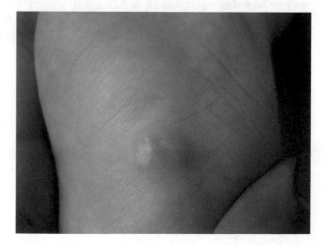

Fig. 9.4 Similar nodule on
the right labia majora.
With permission © 2015
[Sheila Friedlander, M.D.]

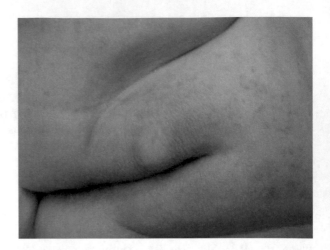

an abdominal mass supports concern for neuroblastoma and also raises concern for
a Wilms tumor with metastasis to the skin.

The next step should be a biopsy of the lesion and imaging of the abdominal
mass.

Biopsy showed dermis filled with a monomorphic population of small blue cells
with a high nuclear-to-cytoplasmic ratio and dispersed nuclear chromatin. Focally,
blue cells were formed into rosettes around a clear center (Homer-Wright rosettes).
Scattered mitotic figures and cells with karyorrhexis were seen. Computed tomography (CT) imaging of the chest, abdomen, and pelvis showed a large mass
(10×6×8.5 cm) in the left lower abdomen, which encased the intra-abdominal
great vessels and appeared to arise from an extra-adrenal location rather than from
the adrenals themselves. Additionally, there was metastatic involvement of the liver
and left paraspinal region.

Metastatic neuroblastoma was diagnosed based on these findings. Further
workup included measurement of LDH, uric acid, HVA and VMA, tumor cytogenetics, magnetic resonance imaging (MRI) of the spine, bone marrow biopsy,
Technetium 99 scan, and metaiodobenzylguanidine (MIBG) scan. HVA and VMA
levels were measured and MIBG scan performed because 90 % of neuroblastomas
secrete catecholamines and take up MIBG [28].

Laboratory Values

- Total bilirubin: 0.8 (0.1–1 mg/dL)
- Direct bilirubin: <0.1 (0.0–0.6 mg/dL)
- LDH: 1301 (550–1000 U/L)

- AST: 81 (20–60 U/L)
- ALT: 28 (5–48 U/L)
- VMA: 580 (<27 μg/mg Cr)
- HVA: 286 (<35 μg/mg Cr)

MRI Spine

Extensive paraspinal spread with multilevel tumor extension but no frank cord compression.

Bone Marrow Biopsy

Normal marrow cellularity for the patient's age (90–95 %). Approximately 50 % of the core is involved by a metastatic neoplasm composed of islands of small blue cells with abundant neuropil formations. The neoplastic cells show a nesting pattern and contain occasional mitotic figures.

A 200 cell differential count revealed:

- Blasts: 1 %
- Promyelocytes: 1 %
- Myelocytes: 5 %
- Bands/metamyelocytes: 25 %
- Segmental neutrophils: <4 %
- Lymphocytes: 52 %
- Eosinophils: 1 %
- Monocytes: 7 %
- Erythroid precursors: 4 %

Cytogenetics

Amplification of the MYCN gene was not observed by FISH analysis.

Tc 99 Scan

Bony metastasis to left parietal bone.

MIBG

Large area of radiotracer uptake in the central abdomen and pelvis. In addition, there are multiple areas of focally increased uptake within the osseous structures involving the posterior calvarium, right proximal humerus, left distal humerus, and multiple areas of the bilateral femurs and tibias. There is also an area of increased uptake in the left supraclavicular region.

Discussion

The patient was diagnosed with intermediate risk stage 4/stage M neuroblastoma.

Neuroblastoma is a tumor composed of primitive cells of the sympathetic nervous system [29]. Approximately half of neuroblastomas develop in the adrenal medulla, but they may arise from sympathetic nervous system tissue in any part of the body, including visceral ganglia or paravertebral sympathetic ganglia [29–31]. They are the second most common solid tumor in children and the most common malignant tumor in infants, accounting for 30–50 % of malignant tumors in newborns [29, 31–35]. The prevalence of neuroblastoma is 1 in 7000 live births, and there are approximately 700 new cases per year in the United States [31]. Most neuroblastomas are diagnosed in children younger than 5 years, but they can also develop in adolescents or adults. Neuroblastoma often metastasizes, and 60 % of affected infants have metastatic disease at diagnosis [33]. Although it most commonly metastasizes to lymph nodes, bone, and bone marrow, some infants have a unique pattern of metastatic spread mainly to the liver and skin [31]. Three percent of all neuroblastoma patients have cutaneous metastases, including ~32 % of those with neonatal neuroblastoma [30, 36]. Skin lesions may be the presenting sign of the disease. Cutaneous metastasis in the neonate often creates a blueberry muffin phenotype, with firm, blue-purple papules and nodules [29, 33, 37]. A distinctive feature of cutaneous neuroblastoma is that when the lesions are rubbed, they initially become erythematous for 2–3 min and then blanch and remain blanched for 30 min to an hour [37]. This distinctive feature may be due to catecholamine release by the tumor cells. Other distinctive manifestations of neuroblastoma include periorbital ecchymoses, referred to as "raccoon eyes," due to metastases to the bones of the orbits; variation in the color of the iris, known as heterochromic irides, due to involvement of the sympathetic branch of the ophthalmic nerve which affects eye color; and Horner's syndrome [29, 36]. Patients often have an abdominal mass, as seen in this case, due to metastasis to the liver and may present with fever or failure to thrive [29].

Neuroblastoma is one of several types of pediatric tumors composed of small, round, blue cells. Most cells are undifferentiated, but some may have neuronal differentiation [31, 33]. Histologically, they may be difficult to distinguish from Ewing's sarcoma, leukemia, lymphoma, peripheral neuroectodermal tumors, rhab-domyosarcoma, and acute mega-karyoblastic leukemia [28, 38]. However, neuro-blastoma cells tend to clump into Homer-Wright rosettes around a clear center, which are not typically seen in other tumor types [36, 39]. Presence of neuropil in the bone marrow biopsy is a clue indicating nervous system tissue [40]. Additionally, on electron microscopy, vesicles containing a homogeneous inclusion, which are thought to be catecholamine granules, may be seen [37].

Immunohistochemical markers have limited value for diagnosing neuroblas-toma. CD65, neuroblastoma 84 (NB84), protein gene product 9.5 (PGP9.5), neuron-specific enolase (NSE), neurofilament protein (NFP), and synaptophysin are often expressed in neuroblastoma but are also expressed in other small round blue cell tumors [33, 38, 41–43]. CD99 and PHOX2B staining can help distinguish neuro-blastomas from other small round blue cell tumors; neuroblastoma is positive for PHOX2B but negative for CD99 [43]. Amplification of the c-myc-related oncogene MYCN on the short arm of chromosome 2 has a prevalence of approximately 22 % and is associated with poor prognosis [31, 33].

Most neuroblastomas are sporadic, but a small subset of patients seems to have a familial predisposition to the disease with autosomal dominant inheritance [31].

Neuroblastoma has a variable course, with the possibility of spontaneous remis-sion or extensive metastasis. Overall, neuroblastoma has the highest rate of sponta-neous regression among all malignant tumors [44]. However, as summarized by Brodeur et al., there seem to be two types of neuroblastoma: a biologically favorable type that develops in infants and a biologically unfavorable type that develops in older patients [31]. The International Neuroblastoma Staging System (INSS) or more recent International Neuroblastoma Risk Group Staging System (INRGSS) is used to stage the disease and determine treatment [45].

Infants with cutaneous metastasis usually fall into INRGSS stage MS, which is defined as metastatic disease in children younger than 18 months with metastases confined to skin, liver and/or bone marrow, and bone marrow involvement limited to less than 10 % of total nucleated cells [29, 45]. This pattern of disease, which is similar to stage 4S under the older staging system, often undergoes spontaneous remission or transformation into a benign ganglioneuroma [31, 36]. Therefore, asymptomatic infants with this pattern typically can be observed without treatment [28, 46]. The 5-year overall survival rate for such patients is 91 % [47]. Children older than 18 months are more likely to have extensive or metastatic disease at the time of diagnosis, with poor prognosis and requiring more aggressive treatment [31]. All patients with MYCN amplification are considered high risk and should be started on an aggressive treatment regimen regardless of age or stage [47]. Chromosome 11q deletion, which negatively affects prognosis, and a hyperdiploid karyotype, which positively affects prognosis, may also be considered in making treatment recommendations.

Treatment

Although most patients with cutaneous metastasis have stage MS (stage 4S) disease, this patient had widely metastatic stage M (stage 4) disease, considered intermediate risk due to absence of MYCN amplification and favorable histology. Chemotherapy with doxorubicin, cyclophosphamide, etoposide, and carboplatin was started immediately, and she received a total of eight courses of chemotherapy. After chemotherapy, there was no bone marrow evidence of disease, and the size of her lesions had decreased significantly. She had no remaining evidence of bony metastases, her liver lesions were no longer MIBG avid, and MIBG uptake elsewhere was diminished. She underwent debulking of her primary tumor, and pathology showed no evidence of active neuroblastoma. She has remained disease free for almost 8 years.

Case 9.3

History

A 6-month-old Hispanic boy is referred to dermatology by his pediatrician for a red, bulbous lump on his right buttock. His parents first noticed "a small bruise" when he was 1 month old. By the age of 2 months, it had grown to the size of a dime and was slightly raised. It continued to grow and became firmer, but the patient did not seem bothered by it. Two days ago, it broke open for the first time, oozing a yellow liquid and blood. Since then it has bled intermittently.

Physical Exam

On examination, the child has a 3.5×2 cm violaceous, exophytic nodule with central erosion and crusting protruding from the right gluteal cleft (Fig. 9.5). There is no palpable pulse or thrill in the stalk of the lesion.

Questions

1. What is your differential diagnosis?
2. What is your next step?

Fig. 9.5 Large, eroded
exophytic nodule on the
right buttock of a
6-month-old male.

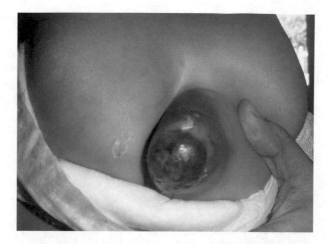

Answers

This rapidly enlarging red, crusted nodule that has begun to bleed might raise concern
for an infantile hemangioma with ulceration. But the continued growth and smooth
yet tense (as opposed to lobular) surface also puts other neoplasms in the differential
diagnosis. These include tufted angioma, kaposiform hemangioendothelioma, rhabdomyosarcoma, myofibroma, and fibrosarcoma [48]. The patient underwent expe-
dited workup, including MRI imaging of the lesion to determine etiology and extent,
and renal and genitourinary ultrasound to assess for features of LUMBAR/PELVIS
syndrome (e.g., genital malformation, lipomyelomeningocele, vesicorenal abnormalities, imperforate anus) which may be associated with infantile hemangioma.

Workup

MRI of the lumbar spine and sacrum with and without contrast showed an approximately 3×4 cm mass within the right gluteal region near the midline. The majority
of the mass was relatively defined; however, there were irregular areas of stranding
surrounding the lesion. The lesion was heterogeneous but primarily T2 hyperin-
tense. The postcontrast images demonstrated irregular nodular and patchy linear
areas of enhancement; however, much of the lesion did not significantly enhance.
This would be unusual for infantile hemangioma as typically they diffusely robustly
enhance and have flow voids.

Ultrasound of kidneys and bladder was normal. Ultrasound of the nodule itself
showed a solid, hypervascular mass with increased flow through the entire lesion.

Given the combination of the MRI and ultrasound findings, an atypical vascular
tumor, such as a non-involuting congenital hemangioma, tufted angioma, or less

likely a kaposiform hemangioma/hemangioendothelioma was considered most likely, but soft tissue sarcoma could not be excluded.

Since the diagnosis remained uncertain after imaging, an excisional biopsy was performed by plastic surgery. The biopsy showed a dense proliferation of spindle cells in a herringbone pattern, with up to ten mitotic figures per high-power field. There were dilated blood vessels, degenerated areas, and collections of blood within the tumor. The tumor was seen invading associated fat.

Immunohistochemistry

- Vimentin: diffusely positive
- SMA: negative
- Desmin: negative
- S100: negative
- CD34: diffusely positive
- Myogenin: negative

Pathology was most consistent with an infantile fibrosarcoma. However, reverse-transcriptase polymerase chain reaction (PCR) did not identify the typical t(12;15) translocation associated with the ETV6/NTRK3 (neurotrophic tyrosine kinase receptor type 3) fusion gene.

Discussion

Fibrosarcoma is a rare tumor of fibroblast cells with an incidence of five per million infants [49, 50]. After rhabdomyosarcomas, fibrosarcomas are the second most common soft tissue sarcomas in children, but they comprise only 1–2 % of all childhood malignancies [51, 52]. Fibrosarcoma in young children is less aggressive and genetically distinct from that in older children and adults, so it is labeled "infantile fibrosarcoma" [53]. The Pediatric Oncology Group staging system for non-rhabdomyosarcoma soft tissue sarcoma defines infantile fibrosarcoma as occurring in a child 4 years or younger [54, 55]. Approximately half of infantile sarcomas are congenital, and the majority is diagnosed in the first year of life [51, 56, 57]. They most often develop on the distal extremities and typically present as a soft tissue mass. Overlying skin can be tense, shiny, erythematous, or ulcerated. Their consistency varies from soft to firm, and they are often poorly circumscribed. Infantile fibrosarcomas may grow rapidly, in some cases doubling in size in weeks to months. They often invade surrounding fibrofatty or muscular tissue.

It is common for infantile fibrosarcomas to clinically appear similar to hemangiomas or vascular/lymphatic malformations. Even on ultrasound and MRI, these lesions may be difficult to distinguish and there are no MRI findings specific for infantile fibrosarcoma [58]. A tumor that is fully formed at birth may be a congenital infantile fibrosarcoma, other malignant neoplasm, or congenital hemangioma. In this case, the lesion was not fully formed at birth but rather grew quickly after the first month; clinically, it mimicked an infantile hemangioma, but as imaging findings were not consistent with this, histologic examination was warranted.

Histology of infantile fibrosarcoma shows immature spindle-shaped cells with high cellularity and prominent mitotic activity. Cells are sometimes arranged in a characteristic herringbone pattern with intertwining fascicles, but histologic diversity has been noted [59–61]. Vascular clefts, myxoid degeneration, hemorrhagic necrosis, and a focal hemangiopericytomatous vascular pattern may be present [56, 57].

Fibrosarcoma usually stains diffusely positive for vimentin, and may be focally positive for actin [54]. Other markers like CD34 and S-100 protein stain positive only in a minority of cases [62]. The tumors typically are negative for myogenin and for GLUT1, the latter being positive in infantile hemangiomas [63, 64]. Immunohistochemistry may be most useful in ruling out other malignant tumors such as rhabdomyosarcoma. However, 20–30 % of infantile fibrosarcomas stain positive for desmin, muscle-specific actin (MSA), or myogenin [54]. This may make differentiation from rhabdomyosarcoma difficult, in which case ultrastructural analysis is valuable; any striated muscle differentiation would suggest a rhabdomyosarcoma.

Most cases of infantile fibrosarcoma have a t(12;15)(p13;q25) translocation, which results in the ETV6-NTRK3 fusion gene [62]. The translocation is detected in 70–90 % of infantile fibrosarcomas and is also found in mesoblastic nephromas; it has not been identified in adult fibrosarcoma or benign infantile lesions [51, 62, 65]. It has been considered to be associated with favorable prognosis and chemosensitivity, but fatal metastatic disease with the t(12;15)(p13;q25) translocation has been reported [66–68].

Overall, the prognosis for infantile fibrosarcoma is good, with 10-year survival almost 90 % [65]. Only 7–8 % of infantile lesions metastasize, although axial lesions may have higher risk (26 % with metastases in one series of 52 patients) [57, 69, 70]. Lungs and bone are the most common sites of metastasis [51]. Despite the relatively low rate of metastasis, local recurrence is common (43 % in one series of 110 children) and typically occurs within 12 months of initial surgical excision [49, 70]. Older children with adult-type fibrosarcoma have higher rates of metastasis (50 % at 5-year follow-up) [65, 70].

Treatment

Surgical excision is the mainstay of treatment for infantile fibrosarcoma. If the tumor can be completely removed without significant morbidity, primary surgical resection should be performed, without adjuvant chemotherapy or radiation therapy, as adjuvant therapies do not confer a survival benefit [51]. Even when margins are microscopically positive, there is no clear benefit from adjuvant chemotherapy [65]. If surgical excision is not possible without significant morbidity (such as amputation), neoadjuvant chemotherapy should be given prior to attempted excision; this is required in more than 75 % of cases [71]. The typical chemotherapy regimen is vincristine and actinomycin-D [65]. Alkylating agents or anthracycline can be added if response to initial chemotherapy is insufficient [65]. In light of the high risk of recurrence, close follow-up is always required, regardless of the initial treatment. For palpable residual lesions, monthly physical exams with imaging every 3 months have been recommended; more frequent ultrasounds are recommended for non-palpable lesions [51]. If local recurrence occurs, surgical resection should be attempted if possible. If the cancer metastasizes, chemotherapy is required; however, metastatic infantile fibrosarcoma is poorly responsive to chemotherapy. An aggressive chemotherapy regimen such as vincristine/doxorubicin/cyclophosphamide alternated with etoposide/ifosfamide is warranted for metastatic disease [51].

This patient underwent wide local excision with negative margins. Chest CT and bone scan showed no evidence of metastasis, and surveillance with imaging every 3 months was planned. However, within 9 months a 0.5×0.8 cm round enhancing lesion recurred on the buttock, and imaging showed metastases to the lungs and the S5 vertebral body. The cancer proved resistant to two rounds of chemotherapy with vincristine, cyclophosphamide, doxorubicin, and ifosfamide. After an assessment of genomic alterations, he was started on the biologic agent Crizotinib, with some improvement.

Case 9.4

History

A 5-year-old boy presented for evaluation of a non-resolving pink-red bump on his mid back present for 2 years. It had not changed in size recently and was not painful or itchy. It had never bled or leaked fluid. He had no significant medical history, and no one else in the family had a history of a similar lesion.

Physical Exam

On physical exam he had a 9 mm pink-red, firm, well-defined papule on his central mid back (Fig. 9.6). He had no other similar lesions on the remainder of his exam.

Biopsy

Given a broad differential diagnosis, excision under sedation was performed. Pathology showed a proliferation of spindle cells with ovoid nuclei, largely arranged perpendicular to the skin surface. There is a somewhat nodular appearance in the

Fig. 9.6 Pink-red bump on the mid back of a 5-year-old boy, unchanged for 2 years. With permission © 2015 [Sheila Friedlander, M.D.]

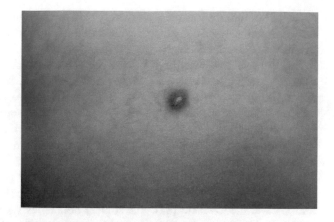

deeper portions of the lesion extending to the lower mid dermis. A grenz zone is identified. A branching "staghorn"-like pattern of blood vessels can be seen between the nodular portions. Mature myoid cells are seen at the periphery. No cytologic atypia or mitotic activity is seen.

Immunohistochemistry

- CD34: lesion essentially negative, except vascular structures positive.
- Factor XIIIa: negative
- Smooth muscle actin (SMA): lesion diffusely positive
- CD68: negative

Questions

1. What is in your differential diagnosis?
2. What workup and treatment is appropriate?

Answers

The differential diagnosis included infantile myofibromatosis, hemangiopericytoma (now considered part of the spectrum of myofibromatosis) [72], and Spitz nevus. Other benign tumors on the differential included dermatofibroma, nodular fasciitis, and desmoid tumor/aggressive fibromatosis. Infantile fibrosarcoma and rhabdomyosarcoma were also considered, although felt to be much less likely given the lack of growth of the lesion. Histologic exam was consistent with a myofibroma.

Infantile myofibromatosis, previously called congenital fibromatosis, is a disorder of myofibroblastic proliferation and one of the most common benign fibrous tumors of infancy, accounting for 12% of pediatric soft tissue tumors [73–75]. It typically presents as discrete, firm or rubbery, flesh-colored, purple, or red nodule(s) ranging in size from less than 1 cm to more than 10 cm. Solitary to multiple lesions (up to 100) have been reported [76, 77]. Dermal nodules may be well defined, while subcutaneous lesions may be poorly demarcated. They sometimes ulcerate and may have telangiectasias or an angiomatous appearance. More than 90% of infantile myofibromatosis appears before 12 months of age, and 76% are congenital [78]. However, it can present later in childhood and, rarely, in adulthood [74, 79–81]. Myofibromas are categorized into three clinical types: (1) solitary cutaneous, (2) multicentric without visceral involvement, and (3) generalized with both cutaneous and visceral involvement [82]. The solitary cutaneous type is most common, comprising 85% of cases in one series of 114 patients [79]. Solitary myofibromas are often found on the head and neck, are painless, and are more common in boys [78–80]. The multicentric and generalized types have no clear gender pattern. Multicentric lesions may be found in subcutaneous tissue, muscle, and bone, as well as skin. The generalized form involves visceral organs in addition to the skin. Up to 57% percent of those with multiple myofibromata have visceral lesions [73, 80, 83]. Although the lesions are benign, they may exert a mass effect, and the generalized form can cause significant visceral dysfunction. The most common sites of visceral involvement are the lungs (51%), gastrointestinal system (47%), heart (37%), and liver (30%) [82]. The condition is usually sporadic but may be inherited in an autosomal dominant fashion [74, 84].

All three forms of myofibromatosis have similar histology, with a two-zone pattern consisting of peripheral fascicles of whorled myoid spindle-shaped cells in a collagen-rich background and central primitive, polygonal cells with a hemangiopericytoma-like pattern [75, 78, 79, 81]. Fibrosis, calcification, and hyalinization may be seen in the center of the lesion. Mitotic rate varies and is not prognostic [75]. Histology typically rules out other conditions on the differential, and immunohistochemistry is confirmatory.

The myofibroblastic cells typically stain positive for smooth muscle actin (SMA) and muscle-specific actin (MSA). Areas with hemangiopericytoma-like vascular pattern stain positive for CD34. In this case, negative staining for CD68 and XIIIA made dermatofibroma less likely [79, 85]. Although nodular fasciitis also stains positive for SMA and MSA, it is more commonly seen in adults [75, 79]. Infantile fibrosarcoma tends to have more uniform spindle cells and often has a t(12;15) translocation, while there is no characteristic chromosomal or molecular marker for myofibromatosis [78, 79].

Infantile myofibromatosis without visceral involvement typically regresses spontaneously within 1–2 years of diagnosis [86]. Nodules may leave atrophic scars or calcification. Hypothesized mechanisms for the spontaneous regression include withdrawal of estrogen after birth, apoptosis, progressive cell differentiation, or factors modulating angiogenesis [74, 87–89]. In some reviews, mortality rates in solitary and multicentric forms without visceral involvement are as low as 0% [73, 82,

90, 91]. Prognosis for the generalized type with visceral involvement is poor due to visceral dysfunction, with mortality at 73–93 % [73, 78].

Although no specific guidelines exist, patients older than 2 years of age with a solitary non-visceral lesion and no signs of multicentric disease generally do not need further workup, as most will not progress [78]. Children younger than two with a solitary lesion should be watched closely for the development of multicentric disease [78]. Some clinicians recommend screening all patients with multiple skin and/or subcutaneous lesions for visceral, soft tissue, and osseous involvement [82, 87]. Abdominal ultrasound, chest X-ray, skeletal survey, CT or MRI of chest and abdomen, and echocardiogram may be considered [78, 87, 92].

Treatment

With high likelihood of spontaneous regression, watchful waiting is preferred to treatment whenever possible [86]. Symptomatic, easily accessible lesions can be surgically excised, but there is a risk of recurrence, with 7 % recurring in one review [80].

No guidelines exist for the treatment of generalized infantile myofibromatosis. Low-intensity chemotherapy has been used successfully in a handful of cases [82]. Methotrexate with vinblastine is the most commonly used chemotherapy treatment and appears to be most effective (8 of 8 patients surviving in one review), but tamoxifen, actinomycin D, cyclophosphamide, prednisolone, interferon-α, and 20-chlorodeoxyadenosine have also been used (43 % survival for these regimens combined) [82].

References

1. Handler MZ, Schwartz RA. Neonatal leukaemia cutis. J Eur Acad Dermatol Venereol. 2015;29(10):1884–9.
2. Gottesfeld E, Silverman RA, Coccia PF, Jacobs G, Zaim MT. Transient blueberry muffin appearance of a newborn with congenital monoblastic leukemia. J Am Dermatol. 1989;21(2 Pt 2):347–51.
3. Zhang IH, Zane LT, Braun BS, Maize J, Zoger S. Congenital leukemia cutis with subsequent development of leukemia. J Am Acad Dermatol. 2006;54(2 Suppl):S22–7.
4. Resnik KS, Brod BB. Leukemia cutis in congenital leukemia: analysis and review of the world literature with report of an additional case. Arch Dermatol. 1993;129(10):1301–6.
5. Choi JH, Lee HB, Park CW, Lee CH. A case of congenital leukemia cutis. Ann Dermatol. 2009;21(1):66–70.
6. Cho-Vega JH, Medeiros LJ, Prieto VG, Vega F. Leukemia cutis. Am J Clin Pathol. 2008;129(1):130–42.
7. Aboutalebi A, Korman JB, Sohani AR, Hasserjian RP, Louissaint Jr A, Le L, et al. Aleukemic cutaneous myeloid sarcoma. J Cutan Pathol. 2013;40(12):996–1005.
8. Paller AS, Mancini AJ. Histiocytoses and malignant skin diseases. In: Paller AS, Mancini AJ, editors. Hurwitz clinical pediatric dermatology. 4th ed. Philadelphia: Elsevier Saunders; 2011. p. 228–9.

9. Boggs DR, Wintrobe MM, Cartwright GE. The acute leukemias. Analysis of 322 cases and review of the literature. Medicine (Baltimore). 1962;41:163–225.

10. Agis H, Weltermann A, Fonatsch C, Haas O, Mitterbauer G, Müllauer L, et al. A comparative study on demographic, hematological, and cytogenetic findings and prognosis in acute myeloid leukemia with and without leukemia cutis. Ann Hematol. 2002;81(2):90–5.

11. Reinhardt D, Creutzig U. Isolated myelosarcoma in children—update and review. Leuk Lymphoma. 2002;43(3):565–74.

12. Su W, Buechner SA, Li CY. Clinicopathologic correlations in leukemia cutis. J Am Acad Dermatol. 1984;11(1):121–8.

13. Sisack MJ, Dunsmore K, Sidhu-Malik N. Granulocytic sarcoma in the absence of myeloid leukemia. J Am Acad Dermatol. 1997;37(2 Pt 2):308–11.

14. Straus DJ, Mertelsmann R, Koziner B, McKenzie S, de Harven E, Arlin ZA, et al. The acute monocytic leukemias: multidisciplinary studies in 45 patients. Medicine (Baltimore). 1980;59(6):409–25.

15. Bresters D, Reus ACW, Veerman AJP, van Wering ER, van der Does-van den Berg A, Kaspers GJL. Congenital leukaemia: the Dutch experience and review of the literature. Br J Haematol. 2002;117(3):513–24.

16. Paydas S, Zorludemir S. Leukaemia cutis and leukaemic vasculitis. Br J Dermatol. 2001;143(4):773–9.

17. Kaddu S, Zenahlik P, Beham-Schmid C, Kerl H, Cerroni L. Specific cutaneous infiltrates in patients with myelogenous leukemia: a clinicopathologic study of 26 patients with assessment of diagnostic criteria. J Am Dermatol. 1999;40(6):966–78.

18. Grundy RG, Martinez A, Kempski H, Malone M, Atherton D. Spontaneous remission of congenital leukemia: a case for conservative treatment. J Pediatr Hematol Oncol. 2000;22(3):252–5.

19. Cronin DMP, George TI, Sundram UN. An updated approach to the diagnosis of myeloid leukemia cutis. Am J Clin Pathol. 2009;132(1):101–10.

20. Buechner SA, Li C-Y, Daniel Su WP, Hunter JAA, Holubar K. Leukemia cutis. A histopathologic study of 42 cases. Am J Dermatopathol. 1985;7(2):109–20.

21. Dabbs DJ. Diagnostic immunohistochemistry. 4th ed. Philadelphia: Elsevier Sciences; 2013. p 488.

22. Fender AB, Gust A, Wang N, Scott GA, Mercurio MG. Congenital leukemia cutis. Pediatr Dermatol. 2008;25(1):34–7.

23. Dinulos JG, Hawkins DS, Clark BS, Francis JS. Spontaneous remission of congenital leukemia. J Pediatr. 1997;131(2):300–3.

24. van der Linden MH, Creemers S, Pieters R. Diagnosis and management of neonatal leukaemia. Semin Fetal Neonatal Med. 2012;17(4):192–5.

25. Balgobind BV, Raimondi SC, Harbott J, Zimmermann M, Alonzo TA, Auvrignon A, et al. Novel prognostic subgroups in childhood 11q23/MLL-rearranged acute myeloid leukemia: results of an international retrospective study. Blood. 2009;114(12):2489–96.

26. Yilmaz Karapinar D, Kamer SA, Karadaş N, Anacak Y, Delcastello BE, Balkan C, et al. Successful treatment with total skin electron beam therapy in a child with isolated cutaneous relapsed AML. J Pediatr Hematol Oncol. 2015;37(6):e372–4.

27. Bakst RL, Tallman MS, Douer D, Yahalom J. How I treat extramedullary acute myeloid leukemia. Blood [Internet]. 2011;118(14):3785–93. http://www.bloodjournal.org/cgi/doi/10.1182/blood-2011-04-347229.

28. Dhir S, Wheeler K. Neonatal neuroblastoma. Early Hum Dev. 2010;86(10):601–5.

29. Paller AS, Mancini AJ, editors. Hurwitz clinical pediatric dermatology. Histiocytosis and malignant skin diseases. 4th ed. Philadelphia: WB Saunders; 2011. p. 232–3.

30. Schneider KM, Becker JM, Krasna IH. Neonatal neuroblastoma. Pediatrics. 1965;36(3P1):359–66.

31. Brodeur GM. Neuroblastoma: biological insights into a clinical enigma. Nat Rev Cancer. 2003;3(3):203–16.

32. Isaacs Jr H. Cutaneous metastases in neonates: a review. Pediatr Dermatol. 2011;28(2): 85–93.
33. Lukens JN. Neuroblastoma in the neonate. Semin Perinatol. 1999;23(4):263–73.
34. Gale GB, D'Angio GJ, Uri A, Chatten J, Koop CE. Cancer in neonates: the experience at the Children's Hospital of Philadelphia. Pediatrics. 1982;70(3):409–13.
35. Campbell AN, Chan HS, O'Brien A, Smith CR, Becker LE. Malignant tumours in the neonate. Arch Dis Child. 1987;62(1):19–23.
36. Lucky AW, McGuire J, Komp DM. Infantile neuroblastoma presenting with cutaneous blanching nodules. J Am Dermatol. 1982;6(3):389–91.
37. Hawthorne HC, Nelson JS, Giangiacomo J, Witzleben CL. Blanching subcutaneous nodules in neonatal neuroblastoma. J Pediatr. 1970;77(2):297–300.
38. Nguyen AV, Argenyi ZB. Cutaneous neuroblastoma. Am J Dermatopathol. 1993;15(1):7–14.
39. van Erp I. Cutaneous metastases in neuroblastoma. Dermatologica. 1968;136(4):265–9.
40. Hicks MJ, Mackay B. Comparison of ultrastructural features among neuroblastic tumors: maturation from neuroblastoma to ganglioneuroma. Ultrastruct Pathol. 1995;19(4):311–22.
41. Cohn SL. Diagnosis and classification of the small round-cell tumors of childhood. Am J Pathol. 1999;155(1):11–5.
42. Wick MR. Immunohistochemical approaches to the diagnosis of undifferentiated malignant tumors. Ann Diagn Pathol. 2008;12(1):72–84.
43. Dabbs DJ. Diagnostic immunohistochemistry. 4th ed. Philadelphia: Elsevier; 2013. p 349–351.
44. Hero B, Simon T, Spitz R, Ernestus K, Gnekow AK, Scheel-Walter HG, et al. Localized infant neuroblastomas often show spontaneous regression: results of the prospective trials NB95-S and NB97. J Clin Oncol. 2008;26(9):1504–10.
45. Monclair T, Brodeur GM, Ambros PF, Brisse HJ, Cecchetto G, Holmes K, et al. The International Neuroblastoma Risk Group (INRG) staging system: an INRG Task Force Report. J Clin Oncol. 2009;27(2):298–303.
46. Nickerson HJ, Matthay KK, Seeger RC, Brodeur GM, Shimada H, Perez C, et al. Favorable biology and outcome of stage IV-S neuroblastoma with supportive care or minimal therapy: a Children's Cancer Group study. J Clin Oncol. 2000;18(3):477–86.
47. Pinto NR, Applebaum MA, Volchenboum SL, Matthay KK, London WB, Ambros PF, et al. Advances in risk classification and treatment strategies for neuroblastoma. J Clin Oncol. 2015;33(27):3008–17.
48. Frieden IJ, Rogers M, Garzon MC. Conditions masquerading as infantile haemangioma: part 1. Australas J Dermatol. 2009;50(2):77–97; quiz 98.
49. Loh ML, Ahn P, Perez-Atayde AR, Gebhardt MC, Shamberger RC, Grier HE. Treatment of infantile fibrosarcoma with chemotherapy and surgery: results from the Dana-Farber Cancer Institute and Children's Hospital, Boston. J Pediatr Hematol Oncol. 2002;24(9):722–6.
50. Ries L, Smith MA, Gurney JG, Linet M, editors. Cancer incidence and survival among children and adolescents: United States SEER Program 1975-1995. National Cancer Institute, SEER Program. NIH Pub. No. 99-4649, Bethesda; 1999.
51. Ferguson WS. Advances in the adjuvant treatment of infantile fibrosarcoma. Expert Rev Anticancer Ther. 2003;3(2):185–91.
52. Miller RW, Young JL, Novakovic B. Childhood cancer. Cancer. 1995;75(1):395–405.
53. Dabbs DJ. Diagnostic immunohistochemistry. 4th ed. Philadelphia: Elsevier; 2013. p 107.
54. Okcu MF, Pappo AS, Hicks J. The nonrhabdomyosarcoma soft tissue sarcomas. In: Pizzo PA, Poplack DG, editors. Principles and practice of pediatric oncology. 6th ed. Philadelphia: Lippincott Williams & Wilkins; 2011. p. 976–7.
55. Khoury JD, Coffin CM, Spunt SL, Anderson JR, Meyer WH, Parham DM. Grading of non-rhabdomyosarcoma soft tissue sarcoma in children and adolescents. Cancer. 2010;116(9):2266–74.
56. Coffin CM, Jaszcz W, O'Shea PA, Dehner LP. So-called congenital-infantile fibrosarcoma: does it exist and what is it? Pediatr Pathol. 1994;14(1):133–50.

57. Chung EB, Enzinger FM. Infantile fibrosarcoma. Cancer. 1976;38(2):729–39.
58. Ainsworth KE, Chavhan GB, Gupta AA, Hopyan S, Taylor G. Congenital infantile fibrosarcoma: review of imaging features. Pediatr Radiol. 2014;44(9):1124–9.
59. Balsaver AM, Butler JJ, Martin RG. Congenital fibrosarcoma. Cancer. 1967;20(10):1607–16.
60. Teo HEL, Peh WCG. A 7-week-old female infant with a left thigh swelling. Am J Orthop. 2003;32(10):513–5.
61. Hu Z, Chou PM, Jennings LJ, Arva NC. Infantile fibrosarcoma—a clinical and histologic mimicker of vascular malformations: case report and review of the literature. Pediatr Dev Pathol. 2013;16(5):357–63.
62. Bourgeois JM, Knezevich SR, Mathers JA, Sorensen PH. Molecular detection of the ETV6-NTRK3 gene fusion differentiates congenital fibrosarcoma from other childhood spindle cell tumors. Am J Surg Pathol. 2000;24(7):937–46.
63. Cessna MH, Zhou H, Perkins SL, Tripp SR, Layfield L, Daines C, et al. Are myogenin and myoD1 expression specific for rhabdomyosarcoma? A study of 150 cases, with emphasis on spindle cell mimics. Am J Surg Pathol. 2001;25(9):1150–7.
64. Yan AC, Chamlin SL, Liang MG, Hoffman B, Attiyeh EF, Chang B, et al. Congenital infantile fibrosarcoma: a masquerader of ulcerated hemangioma. Pediatr Dermatol. 2006;23(4):330–4.
65. Orbach D, Rey A, Cecchetto G, Oberlin O, Casanova M, Thebaud E, et al. Infantile fibrosarcoma: management based on the European experience. J Clin Oncol. 2010;28(2):318–23.
66. McCahon E, Sorensen PHB, Davis JH, Rogers PCJ, Schultz KR. Non-resectable congenital tumors with the ETV6-NTRK3 gene fusion are highly responsive to chemotherapy. Med Pediatr Oncol. 2003;40(5):288–92.
67. Punnett HH, Tomczak EZ, Pawel BR, de Chadarevian JP, Sorensen PH. ETV6-NTRK3 gene fusion in metastasizing congenital fibrosarcoma. Med Pediatr Oncol. 2000;35(2):137–9.
68. Shah NN, Price MR, Loeb DM. Cardiac metastasis and hypertrophic osteoarthropathy in recurrent infantile fibrosarcoma. Pediatr Blood Cancer. 2011;59(1):179–81.
69. Blocker S, Koenig J, Ternberg J. Congenital fibrosarcoma. J Pediatr Surg. 1987;22(7):665–70.
70. Soule EH, Pritchard DJ. Fibrosarcoma in infants and children: a review of 110 cases. Cancer. 1977;40(4):1711–21.
71. Ferrari A, Orbach D, Sultan I, Casanova M, Bisogno G. Neonatal soft tissue sarcomas. Semin Fetal Neonatal Med. 2012;17(4):231–8.
72. Iwafuchi H, Tsuzuki T, Ito R, Miyake H, Okita H, Hamazaki M. Generalized infantile myofibromatosis with a monophasic primitive pattern. Pathol Int. 2015;65(8):432–7.
73. Wiswell TE, Davis J, Cunningham BE, Solenberger R, Thomas PJ. Infantile myofibromatosis: the most common fibrous tumor of infancy. J Pediatr Surg. 1988;23(4):314–8.
74. Mashiah J, Hadj-Rabia S, Dompmartin A, Harroche A, Laloum-Grynberg E, Wolter M, et al. Infantile myofibromatosis: a series of 28 cases. J Am Acad Dermatol. 2014;71(2):264–70.
75. Coffin CM, Alaggio R. Fibroblastic and myofibroblastic tumors in children and adolescents. Pediatr Dev Pathol. 2012;15 Suppl 1:127–80. http://www.pedpath.org/doi/abs/10.2350/10-12-0944-PB.1.
76. Goldberg NS, Bauer BS, Kraus H, Crussi FG, Esterly NB. Infantile myofibromatosis: a review of clinicopathology with perspectives on new treatment choices. Pediatr Dermatol. 1988;5(1):37–46.
77. Brill PW, Yandow DR, Langer LO, Breed AL, Laxova R, Gilbert EF. Congenital generalized fibromatosis. Case report and literature review. Pediatr Radiol. 1982;12(6):269–78.
78. Matthews MR, Cockerell CJ. An historic perspective of infantile myofibromatosis. Adv Dermatol. 2006;22:279–305.
79. Oudijk L, den Bakker MA, Hop WCJ, Cohen M, Charles AK, Alaggio R, et al. Solitary, multifocal and generalized myofibromas: clinicopathological and immunohistochemical features of 114 cases. Histopathology. 2012;60(6B):E1–11.
80. Chung EB, Enzinger FM. Infantile myofibromatosis. Cancer. 1981;48(8):1807–18.
81. Hogan SF, Salassa JR. Recurrent adult myofibromatosis. A case report. Am J Clin Pathol. 1992;97(6):810–4.

82. Wu SY, McCavit TL, Cederberg K, Galindo RL, Leavey PJ. Chemotherapy for generalized infantile myofibromatosis with visceral involvement. J Pediatr Hematol Oncol. 2015;37(5): 402–5.
83. Kauffman SL, Stout AP. Congenital mesenchymal tumors. Cancer. 1965;18:460–76.
84. Smith A, Orchard D. Infantile myofibromatosis: two families supporting autosomal dominant inheritance. Australas J Dermatol. 2011;52(3):214–7.
85. Mentzel T, Kutzner H, Rütten A, Hügel H. Benign fibrous histiocytoma (dermatofibroma) of the face: clinicopathologic and immunohistochemical study of 34 cases associated with an aggressive clinical course. Am J Dermatopathol. 2001;23(5):419–26.
86. Schrodt BJ, Callen JP. A case of congenital multiple myofibromatosis developing in an infant. Pediatrics. 1999;104(1 Pt 1):113–5.
87. Wiswell TE, Sakas EL, Stephenson SR, Lesica JJ, Reddoch SR. Infantile myofibromatosis. Pediatrics. 1985;76(6):981–4.
88. Benjamin SP, Mercer RD, Hawk WA. Myofibroblastic contraction in spontaneous regression of multiple congenital mesenchymal hamartomas. Cancer. 1977;40(5):2343–52.
89. Hatzidaki E, Korakaki E, Voloudaki A, Daskaloyannaki M, Manoura A, Giannakopoulou C. Infantile myofibromatosis with visceral involvement and complete spontaneous regression. J Dermatol. 2001;28(7):379–82.
90. Baer JW, Radkowski MA. Congenital multiple fibromatosis. A case report with review of the world literature. Am J Roentgenol Radium Ther Nucl Med. 1973;118(1):200–5.
91. Levine E, Fréneaux P, Schleiermacher G, Brisse H, Pannier S, Teissier N, et al. Risk-adapted therapy for infantile myofibromatosis in children. Pediatr Blood Cancer. 2011;59(1):115–20.
92. Counsell SJ, DeVile C, Mercuri E, Allsop JM, Birch R, Muntoni F. Magnetic resonance imaging assessment of infantile myofibromatosis. Clin Radiol. 2002;57(1):67–70.

Chapter 10
Vascular Anomalies

Sheilagh M. Maguiness and Christina L. Boull

Keywords Infantile hemangioma • Kaposiform hemangioendothelioma • Kasabach–Merritt phenomenon • Localized intravascular coagulopathy • LUMBAR syndrome • Propranolol • Rapidly involuting congenital hemangioma • Sirolimus • Venous malformation • Multifocal lymphangioendotheliomatosis • Glomuvenous malformation • Blue rubber bleb nevus syndrome

Introduction

Vascular anomalies represent a diverse group of entities, each with unique natural history and associated complications. To meet the needs of this challenging population, many referral centers now have interdisciplinary clinics devoted specifically to vascular lesions.

Correct diagnosis is essential to anticipate potential complications and deliver appropriate treatment, and depends on an understanding of the classification of vascular anomalies. The gold-standard classification schema which was first proposed by Mulliken and Glowacki in 1982 is accepted and regularly updated by the International Society for the Study of Vascular Anomalies (ISSVA) [1]. This schema divides vascular anomalies into tumors and malformations based on their biologic characteristics. Vascular tumors such as infantile and congenital hemangiomas often change rapidly in size during the first few weeks to months of life. Vascular malformations such as venous and capillary malformations are fully formed at birth, but gradually enlarge or become more prominent with time. In the first few weeks of life, capillary malformations and infantile hemangiomas may appear very similar on exam, but the presence of bright red islands of proliferation, prominent veins, and detection of elevated blood flow with a bedside doppler (all observed in infantile hemangiomas) are useful ways to distinguish the two.

S.M. Maguiness, MD (✉) • C.L. Boull, MD
Divison of Pediatric Dermatology, Department of Dermatology, University of Minnesota, 420 Delaware St. SE, Minneapolis, MN 55455, USA
e-mail: smaguine@umn.edu; oehr0005@umn.edu

© Springer International Publishing Switzerland 2016   173
M. Hogeling (ed.), *Case-Based Inpatient Pediatric Dermatology*,
DOI 10.1007/978-3-319-31569-0_10

Systemic complications or underlying structural anomalies are uncommon in patients with small, focal vascular lesions, but should be considered when lesions are large, regional/segmental, or multifocal.

The cases described in this chapter represent a small but important sampling of vascular birthmarks in children with associated complications that may present in an inpatient setting.

Case 10.1

History

An otherwise healthy 3-week-old female is seen in the emergency department for evaluation of a large purple nodule on her right posterior shoulder and back. The lesion was present at birth and was stable until 1 day ago when it enlarged and became dark purple. Parents note bruises on the arms and legs that developed over the last day without a history of associated trauma. The infant is feeling well, is afebrile.

Physical Exam

Notable for a purple mass on the right posterior shoulder and back (Fig. 10.1). Scattered purpuric patches are present on the bilateral flexor and extensor upper and lower extremities.

Fig. 10.1 Firm violet and magenta plaque on the right posterior shoulder and back (Photo courtesy of Dr. Kristen Hook)

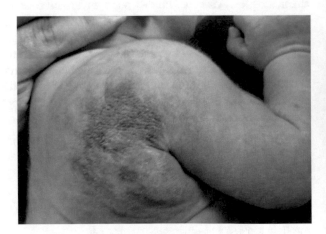

Laboratory Parameters

- Wbc: 5.7 [5.0–14.5 10e9 L⁻¹]
- Hgb: 9.2 [10.5–14.0 g/dL]
- Plt: 28 [150–450 10e9 L⁻¹]
- INR: 2.4 [0.86–1.14]
- PTT: 53 [22–37 s]
- D-dimer: 36.8 [0.0–0.50 µg/mL]
- Fibrinogen activity: 62 [200–420 mg/dL]
- Peripheral smear: consistent with microangiopathic hemolytic anemia with thrombocytopenia and schistocytes

MRI with Contrast

- Ill-defined enhancing soft tissue mass with cutaneous thickening, soft tissue stranding infiltrating multiple tissue planes.
- Multiple flow voids are present within the mass.

Questions

1. What is the diagnosis?
2. What other entities can present with a similar clinical picture?
3. What are the signs and lab abnormalities associated with Kasabach–Merritt Phenomenon?
4. What are possible treatment options?

Answer

Kaposiform hemangioendothelioma (KHE) is a rare vascular tumor presenting shortly after birth or in the first few months of life, and is most commonly located on the trunk or extremities. Up to 10 % may be located internally in the retroperitoneum or intracranially, and show no skin lesions [2]. Clinically, lesions appear as rapidly enlarging singular violet to deep red plaques or nodules. They can be distinguished from infantile hemangiomas by several features. Infantile hemangiomas are less firm to palpation with bright red coloration if superficial, or blue discoloration if deep. Imaging with MRI can aid in diagnosis and will show enhancement with deep tissue involvement, sometimes to the level of bone, with flow voids representing intralesional vascular channels [2–6].

KHE most commonly presents with associated Kasabach–Merritt phenomenon (KMP), a life-threatening consumptive coagulopathy produced by platelet trapping within the vascular tumor [2]. Signs of KMP include rapid enlargement of the vascular tumor with overlying expanding purpura. Laboratory studies for bleeding diathesis will show thrombocytopenia, anemia, elevated D-dimer and fibrin split products, low fibrinogen, and prolonged aPTT and PT. Schistocytes may be noted on a peripheral smear [2, 6–8]. As a result of KMP the patient may develop increased bleeding in the form of hematuria, hematochezia, or diffuse ecchymoses. Infantile hemangiomas, previously thought to be associated with KMP, are now known to be only rarely associated with coagulopathies [4, 5]. Tufted angioma, a vascular tumor of infancy which may in fact represent a clinical variant of KHE [3] can also produce KMP, but is less commonly associated than KHE. All KHE can produce KMP, but it is less common in lesions less than 8 cm in diameter [7].

Treatment

Treatment of KHE is challenging and requires a multi-specialty approach. Past treatment modalities employed with variable success have included systemic steroids, interferon alpha, embolization, radiotherapy, and various chemotherapeutic regimens. In a consensus-derived treatment protocol [3], initial treatment for KHE without KMP is monotherapy with systemic steroids. In the setting of KMP, vincristine, a vinca alkaloid chemotherapeutic agent, should be added. With successful treatment platelet numbers and clotting measures should improve within 4 weeks. A more recent review of KMP suggests that surgical resection or arterial embolization should be considered in small or amenable lesions [8]. In non-bleeding lesions, the addition of combination antiplatelet therapy with aspirin and ticlopidine may have added benefit to other systemic treatments without increasing the bleeding risk [9].

Per consensus conference recommendations, platelet transfusions should only be given during active bleeding or immediately prior to surgery, as increased platelet activation will worsen the consumptive coagulopathy. Fresh frozen plasma, cryoprecipitate, or fibrinogen concentrate are preferred in the setting of active bleeding or fibrinogen levels <1 g/L. Heparin must be avoided as it increases bleeding risk [3].

Multiple small case reports have described KHEs, refractory to multiple treatments, that have responded rapidly to systemic sirolimus [10, 11], an inhibitor of the PI3/AKT/mTOR pathway. Sirolimus is currently a second-line treatment option, but further studies may elevate its status in the treatment ladder.

Case 10.2. Venous Malformation

History

A 12-month-old male presents to the emergency department with acute onset leg pain and swelling. His mother reports that he stumbled while walking, falling onto the right thigh and buttocks. Within a few hours his right thigh began to swell and

Fig. 10.2 Purple patch overlying the buttocks, thigh, calf with associated fullness to the underlying soft tissues

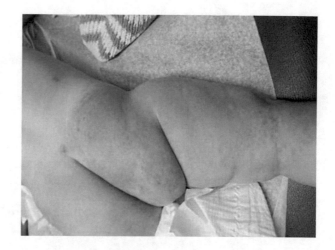

the child refused to walk. He has no associated bruising. Since birth the patient has had increased fullness of the tissues of the right leg with multiple overlying purple plaques. They become larger when he is standing or crying.

Physical Exam

The diameter of the right leg is larger than the left from the level of the thigh to the ankle. There is no limb length discrepancy. There are purple plaques containing dilated vessels on the right buttocks, the upper inner thigh and over the right dorsal foot (Fig. 10.2). Bedside doppler is negative for pulsatile flow within the vascular plaques. The child cries with palpation of the right upper thigh.

Laboratory Parameters

- Wbc: 6.6 [5.0–14.5 10e9 L⁻¹]
- Hgb: 12.2 [10.5–14.0 g/dL]
- Plt: 120 [150–450 10e9 L⁻¹]
- INR: 1.1 [0.86–1.14]
- aPTT: 24 [22–37 s]
- D-dimer: 2.8 [0.0–0.50 µg/mL]
- Fibrinogen activity: 202 [200–420 mg/dL]

X-ray of Lower Extremity

- Soft tissue thickening with scattered calcified phlebolith.
- No bony changes.

Questions

1. What are the natural history/growth characteristics for simple Venous Malformations?
2. What further imaging test(s) are recommended?
3. What lab abnormalities would you expect?
4. What are the risk factors for coagulopathy in the setting of a Venous Malformation?
5. Are there measures you can recommend to prevent future similar episodes?

Answer

Venous malformations (VM) are the most common of the vascular malformations [12]. They present as compressible blue nodules, most commonly on an extremity, and are often associated with prominent dilation of surrounding veins. Deep malformations may infiltrate muscle or viscera and only a subcutaneous fullness or asymmetry may be noted [6]. Crying, Valsalva, and gravity will increase the size of VMs. In contrast to vascular proliferations such as infantile hemangiomas, VMs have slow blood flow and are present fully formed at birth. They are most often diagnosed in the first weeks of life, but are also the most likely vascular anomaly to be diagnosed after the age of 10 [13]. They are also often misdiagnosed as other types of vascular anomalies. Less than half of patients with VMs seen in a specialized vascular lesions clinics had a correct diagnosis prior to referral [12]. MRI with and without contrast is the imaging test of choice to distinguish VMs from other vascular lesions.

In contrast to vascular proliferations that have a rapid growth phase, most venous malformations grow in proportion to the affected child. Large or multifocal lesions, especially when located on the trunk or extremities, are more likely to have a progressive nature. They may become more bulky or prominently dilated over time and result in bony abnormalities, limb length discrepancy, and disfigurement. Hormonal stimulation of VEGF expression and endothelial proliferation, especially during adolescence and pregnancy increase the risk for progression or worsening [14]. Treatment of VM may include observation, compression garments, low-dose aspirin, sclerotherapy, or surgery. Almost all patients with venous malformation experience associated pain [15]. Chronic pain may be produced by many factors including compression of adjacent tendons and nerves, venous insufficiency, and intraosseous or joint involvement [16]. Two triggers for pain due to abnormal clotting are localized intravascular coagulation (LIC) and deep venous thrombosis which require more immediate attention.

Venous malformations, especially those that are large, intramuscular, or contain phleboliths, produce a unique type of LIC due to venous stasis, without systemic symptoms [17]. This differs from the generalized consumptive coagulopathy seen in Kasabach–Merritt phenomenon. Patients with recurrent episodes of acute pain are more likely to have elevated D-dimer levels, a sensitive marker for LIC [16, 17]. During times of trauma or surgical resection, LIC may progress to widespread consumptive coagulopathy in the form of disseminated intravascular coagulation (DIC). This can be distinguished from LIC by elevation of PT and decreased fibrinogen and platelets in conjunction with high D-dimer. Patients will also show evidence of hemolytic anemia on peripheral smear. Bleeding complications may be severe [16].

Deep venous thrombosis is another serious cause of acute pain in venous malformation. Previously described mainly in the setting of Klippel–Trenaunay syndrome, recent data suggests that those with large VMs may also develop clots with potential for pulmonary embolism. A group of patients with VMs with >15 % body surface area involvement were found to have significantly higher pulmonary artery systolic pressures than matched controls. Pulmonary artery pressure correlated with D-dimer levels, suggesting that clots within the venous malformations were producing pulmonary emboli and associated pulmonary hypertension [18].

Treatment

In children with large venous malformations and elevated D-dimer or frequent pain episodes, low-dose aspirin is a safe and effective treatment. Children with VMs treated with aspirin at a dose of 5–10 mg/kg/day had decreased pain and swelling. The main side effect was non-life-threatening bruising or bleeding episodes (e.g., epistaxis, heavy menses). The authors note that complications of gastrointestinal bleeding and Reye's syndrome occur with only much higher aspirin doses, and that there have been no reports of Reye's in children taking low-dose aspirin. Compression garments are another important treatment adjunct, anecdotally reported to decrease pain. They may prevent clotting by minimizing venous stasis in dilated vessels [19–21].

The risk of progression of localized LIC to DIC is particularly high in the setting of surgery. For children with large VMs, elevated D-dimer, and low fibrinogen, pre- and postsurgical courses of low molecular weight heparin are recommended [16].

Case 10.3. LUMBAR Syndrome

History

A 3-week-old newborn with a birthmark over the sacrum and buttocks presents with associated pain and peri-anal bleeding. The infant was born at 36 weeks gestation due to premature rupture of membranes, but has been otherwise healthy. The birthmark has grown rapidly over the last 2 weeks, and has formed an open sore centrally. The infant cries with diaper changes and seems to be in pain.

Fig. 10.3 Reticulated red patch with overlying vascular papules and plaques extending into the gluteal cleft

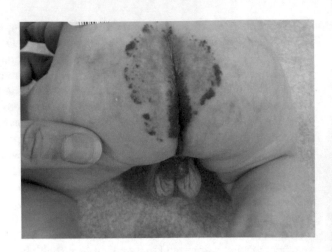

Physical Exam

Skin exam is notable for a large reticulated pink patch overlying the sacrum and bilateral buttocks with extension into the gluteal cleft (Fig. 10.3). There are overlying small venules. By bedside doppler you hear loud pulsation within the lesion. There are no sacral pits or deviation of the spine. There is an ulceration present centrally within the gluteal cleft and peri-anal area with a surrounding rim of pallor.

Questions

1. What imaging tests are recommended?
2. What is the most common associated anomaly?
3. Compared to other infantile hemangiomas, what is the risk of ulceration in this location?
4. What are the treatment options in the setting of ulceration?
5. What is the systemic treatment of choice and recommended dosing?
6. What are the most common side effects and most serious potential side effects of systemic treatment?

Answer

Infantile hemangiomas (IH), when presenting in a segmental distribution should trigger suspicion for associated complications [22]. Segmental IHs in the diaper area may be difficult to recognize and are often initially misdiagnosed as capillary malformations, diaper rash, or erosions and ulcerations [23, 24]. In this location, a disproportionate number of IHs may display a "minimal growth" pattern and fail to proliferate as expected [23]. Clinicians may observe only a pink reticulated patch as opposed to the bright red vascular plaques seen in classic IHs. The finding of high blood flow with bedside doppler is very helpful in the diagnosis of IH.

The specific constellation of findings associated with segmental IHs in the diaper area is known as LUMBAR syndrome (Lower body infantile hemangioma, Urogenital anomalies, ulceration, Myelopathy, Bony deformities, Anorectal anomalies, arterial anomalies, and Renal anomalies) [24]. The same entity has also been reported in the literature as SACRAL and PELVIS syndromes [25, 26]. Most patients will not display all associated findings. The most common extracutaneous association was tethered spinal cord seen in 57 % of patients [27]. The risk of underlying anomalies varies by the specific territory covered by the IH, with those localized to the posterior buttocks more likely to be associated with urogenital, anorectal, and renal abnormalities. Those overlying lower limbs may produce arterial anomalies and associated limb atrophy [27].

Specific imaging recommendations are based on the site of the IH. In infants younger than 3 months of age initial imaging should include ultrasound of the spine, abdomen, and pelvis with Doppler. For children older than 3 months with IH over the lumbosacral spine, an adjunct MRI is recommended, even in the setting of a negative US, due to the high risk of a tethered cord [27–29]. In a prospective study of children with IH >2.5 cm in diameter overlying the midline lumbar or sacral spine, 51 % of patient were found to have an underlying spinal abnormality. The sensitivity for ultrasound detection of these was poor at 50 % [28].

Perineal IHs are at an increased risk of ulceration compared to other IHs. In one series, 45 % of patients with perineal IHs had ulceration at the time of presentation [30]. Central white pallor is a warning sign of impending ulceration [31]. Once ulcerated, hemangiomas are extremely painful and are at increased risk of scarring. Complications of ulceration specific to scarring in the diaper area include deformity or functional deficits of the rectum or genitals. Topical treatment adjuncts such as liberal use of petrolatum-based emollients, 2–5 % lidocaine ointment, metronidazole cream, and non-adherent wound dressing may help to decrease pain and promote healing [32]. Topical timolol may also help to expedite healing [33]. The early introduction of systemic propranolol may halt proliferation and prevent ulceration [30, 34]. In a retrospective cohort study of children with genitourinary or perineal IH, those seen in the pre-propranolol era (prior to 2009) had higher rates of ulceration compared to those treated after 2009 [29].

A recent randomized controlled trial investigating the optimal duration and dosing of oral propranolol for IH found that a dose of 3 mg/kg/day for 6 months duration produced the best clinical outcomes [35]. Potential complications of propranolol therapy include hypotension and bradycardia, but these adverse effects are rare, experienced by <1 % of infants in a large systematic review [36]. Even at the higher dose of 3 mg/kg/day, there was no increase in serious adverse events in treated infants compared to the placebo group [35]. In infants with LUMBAR with IHs overlying a lower extremity, imaging of leg vasculature is recommended to ensure that there is not severe arterial stenosis that could be exacerbated by propranolol [27].

Case 10.4

History

You are called to the neonatal intensive care unit to assess a 1-day-old infant with a large nodule on the leg. The child is full term and had a normal spontaneous vaginal delivery. There were no complications during pregnancy. Apgars were 8 and 9 at 1 and 5 min. Vital signs have remained normal. The lesion has not bled and the infant does not seem in pain with palpation to the area.

Physical Exam

Normal faces. Normal tone. No hepatosplenomegaly. Flat fontanelles. The right thigh shows a 6 cm purple flat-topped nodule with a rim of blanching on the surrounding skin (Fig. 10.4). There are central telangiectasias. There are no other similar lesions.

Fig. 10.4 Telangiectatic plaque with overlying dilated venules and hyporemic rim

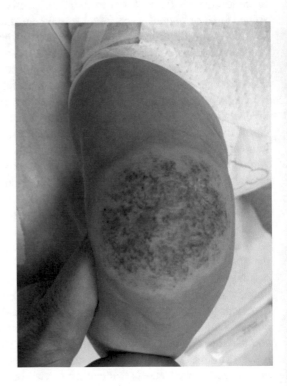

Laboratory Parameters

- Wbc: 12.3 [5.0–14.5 10e9 L^{-1}]
- Hgb: 13.8 [10.5–14.0 g/dL]
- Plt: 82 [150–450 10e9 L^{-1}]
- INR: 0.9 [0.86–1.14]
- aPTT: 30 [22–37 s]

Imaging

- Hypoechoic subcutaneous mass containing tubular vascular structures with mixed, but predominantly venous flow signal.

Questions

1. How would you counsel parents about the progression of this lesion?
2. How can you differentiate this lesion from other congenital vascular proliferations on exam?
3. What are the histopathologic and immunohistochemical features of this tumor?
4. If this lesion were localized to the liver, what would be the potential complications?

Answer

The history and exam suggests a diagnosis of rapidly involuting congenital hemangioma (RICH). Congenital hemangiomas (CH) differ from infantile hemangiomas (IH) as CH are fully formed at birth. They do not exhibit a postnatal proliferation phase, but rather proliferate in utero. On exam, RICH, and its counterpart NICH (non-involuting congenital hemangioma), present as solitary violaceous nodules with overlying telangiectasia or fine venules and a surrounding white halo. Some will have a soft central depression or ulceration. In one series, the mean diameter was 6 cm, but they may be considerably larger. RICH are most commonly located on the head, neck, or extremities [37–39].

RICH and NICH have similar clinical and histological morphology and are distinguished by the presence or absence of involution, respectively. RICH that begin to involute, but then halt and stabilize in size are described as PICH (partially involuting congenital hemangiomas) [40]. RICH involute completely within 6–14 months of life, and may begin their involution phase in utero [41]. RICH, NICH, and IH all demonstrate high flow by bedside doppler which decreases with involution [42]. Histologically RICH are composed of capillary lobules with endothelial cells and pericytes surrounded by fibrous tissue.

Central involution may be noted. Thrombosis, cyst formation, calcification, and extramedullary hematopoiesis are also described. Neither RICH nor NICH express glucose transporter-1 protein (GLUT-1) which is unique to IH [39] and helpful in differentiating the two.

RICHs are occasionally identified on routine prenatal ultrasounds, usually in the second trimester [41, 43, 44]. They may fully involute prior to birth, leaving behind a pale atrophic plaque with dilated veins [42]. Residual fibrofatty tissue changes are absent in involuted RICH, but are common in involuted IHs. While most RICH require no treatment, NICH and PICH require excision if they are cosmetically or functionally problematic. In rare instances ulcerated RICH have bled severely, and in this situation percutaneous embolization is the treatment of choice [45].

RICH may also arise in the liver, usually in the absence of cutaneous lesions. Hepatic RICH are solitary. They are differentiated from the multifocal or diffuse hepatic IH of infantile hemangiomatosis where multiple cutaneous IH are also present [46–48]. Hepatic RICH may be discovered on prenatal ultrasound, or may become symptomatic within the first few months of life with a triad of hepatomegaly, high-output heart failure, and anemia [49]. Heart failure results from high-flow hepatic arteriovenous or portovenous shunts that, in combination with the high blood flow demands of the hemangioma, produce a steal phenomenon. Low-grade anemia and thrombocytopenia are caused by intralesional thrombosis [47]. Other common lab abnormalities include elevated bilirubin and lactate dehydrogenase. Cases of severe transaminitis with liver failure have been reported, but this finding is very rare [50]. Hepatic RICH involute quickly and asymptomatic lesions may be simply observed [48]. In the setting of heart failure or liver failure, treatment is needed. RICH, unlike IH, do not respond to systemic propranolol. First-line treatment includes medical management with corticosteroids. If the response is not adequate, percutaneous embolization of shunts should be considered [47, 48].

Case 10.5. Multifocal Vascular Lesions

History

This 8-week-old infant is seen in the Emergency room for numerous violaceous birthmarks and recent GI bleeding. She was born at full term without any prenatal or postnatal complications. The family states that the infant has had the skin lesions since birth. There is no family history of similar skin lesions in the parents, or other family members. The infant has two healthy siblings. On clinical examination you note numerous violaceous vascular papules and plaques randomly distributed throughout the body (Fig. 10.5).

Fig. 10.5 Multiple
violaceous papules and
plaques over the trunk and
extremities (Photo courtesy
of Beth Drolet, MD)

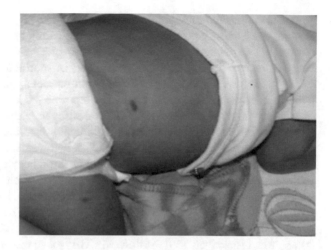

Laboratory Findings

- Hemoglobin 8 g/dL (10.5–14 g/dL)
- Platelet count 58 (150–450 10e9 L^{-1})
- D-dimer 6.1, (<1)
- Fibrinogen, INR, PTT were normal

Questions

1. What is your differential diagnosis for multifocal vascular birthmarks?
2. What are the histopathologic features of multifocal lymphangioendotheliomatosis?
3. What are the possible complications associated with multifocal lymphangioendotheliomatosis?

Answer

Multifocal lymphangioendotheliomatosis (MLT), also known as cutaneovisceral angiomatosis, with thrombocytopenia (CAT) is a recently described condition characterized by multifocal vascular lesions [51, 52]. Lesions in MLT are GLUT-1 negative and distinguishable from multifocal infantile hemangiomas which demonstrate GLUT-1 positivity on immunohistochemical staining [51]. MLT presents in the neonatal period with numerous, randomly distributed red-brown, violaceous, or bluish papules and nodules of varying sizes. There are case reports of patients with MLT and sparse or absent cutaneous involvement. Histopathology reveals proliferation of small thin-walled vessels with hobnailed endothelium. Some vessels also demonstrate intraluminal papillary projections and hyalinization of vessel walls. Lesions are typically positive for LYVE-1 indicating probable lymphatic differentiation [51]. Gastrointestinal bleeding due to involvement of the GI tract with similar vascular lesions is the most common cause of morbidity and mortality in these patients. Outside of the skin and GI tract, intracranial, pulmonary, intraperitoneal, and other visceral involvement have been reported [53].

In the differential diagnosis of multifocal vascular lesions presenting in the neonatal period, the most common entity is multifocal infantile hemangiomas. While multifocal IH are associated with extracutaneous involvement, most commonly hepatic hemangiomas, gastrointestinal involvement or thrombocytopenia are quite rare [54]. In the case of multifocal venous malformations (VM) or glomuvenous malformations (GVM), lesions would present as blue-hued, compressible nodules. GI involvement or LIC (localized intravascular coagulopathy) would not be expected but can rarely occur in the setting of blue rubber bleb nevus syndrome (BRBNS) or large/intramuscular VMs, respectively [55]. Multifocal KHEs may present with profound thrombocytopenia in the setting of Kasabach–Merrit phenomenon, however GI involvement would be uncommon. A skin biopsy may be helpful to confirm the diagnosis.

The prognosis and long-term outcomes in patients with MLT are poorly understood, however attempts are being made to further characterize the condition and follow patients, including a patient registry. In the past MLT has been associated with significant morbidity and mortality mainly related to catastrophic hemorrhage. Numerous treatments have been reported with limited success including corticosteroids, alpha interferon, IVIG vincristine, thalidomide, and bevacizumab [56, 57]. Recently the expanded use of sirolimus in the setting of vascular anomalies, particularly those with lymphatic differentiation, has led to use in numerous vascular anomalies conditions. There are promising reports regarding use of sirolimus in MLT [58].

References

1. Mulliken JB, Glowacki J. Classification of pediatric vascular lesions. Plast Reconstr Surg. 1982;70(1):120–1.
2. Croteau SE, Liang MG, Kozakewich HP, Alomari AI, Fishman SJ, Mulliken JB, Trenor 3rd CC. Kaposiform hemangioendothelioma: atypical features and risks of Kasabach-Merritt phenomenon in 107 referrals. J Pediatr. 2013;162(1):142–7.
3. Drolet BA, Trenor 3rd CC, Brandão LR, Chiu YE, Chun RH, Dasgupta R, Garzon MC, Hammill AM, Johnson CM, Tlougan B, Blei F, David M, Elluru R, Frieden IJ, Friedlander SF, Iacobas I, Jensen JN, King DM, Lee MT, Nelson S, Patel M, Pope E, Powell J, Seefeldt M, Siegel DH, Kelly M, Adams DM. Consensus-derived practice standards plan for complicated Kaposiform hemangioendothelioma. J Pediatr. 2013;163(1):285–91.
4. Enjolras O, Wassef M, Mazoyer E, Frieden IJ, Rieu PN, Drouet L, Taïeb A, Stalder JF, Escande JP. Infants with Kasabach-Merritt syndrome do not have "true" hemangiomas. J Pediatr. 1997;130(4):631–40.
5. Sarkar M, Mulliken JB, Kozakewich HP, Robertson RL, Burrows PE. Thrombocytopenic coagulopathy (Kasabach-Merritt phenomenon) is associated with Kaposiform hemangioendothelioma and not with common infantile hemangioma. Plast Reconstr Surg. 1997;100(6):1377–86.

6. Paller AS, Mancini AJ. Hurwitz clinical pediatric dermatology: a textbook of skin disorders of childhood and adolescence. Philadelphia: Elsevier; 2011.
7. Gruman A, Liang MG, Mulliken JB, Fishman SJ, Burrows PE, Kozakewich HP, Blei F, Frieden IJ. Kaposiform hemangioendothelioma without Kasabach-Merritt phenomenon. J Am Acad Dermatol. 2005;52(4):616–22.
8. O'Rafferty C, O'Regan GM, Irvine AD, Smith OP. Recent advances in the pathobiology and management of Kasabach-Merritt phenomenon. Br J Haematol. 2015;171(1):38–51.
9. Osio A, Fraitag S, Hadj-Rabia S, Bodemer C, de Prost Y, Hamel-Teillac D. Clinical spectrum of tufted angiomas in childhood: a report of 13 cases and a review of the literature. Arch Dermatol. 2010;146(7):758–63.
10. Kai L, Wang Z, Yao W, Dong K, Xiao X. Sirolimus, a promising treatment for refractory Kaposiform hemangioendothelioma. J Cancer Res Clin Oncol. 2014;140(3):471–6.
11. Blatt J, Stavas J, Moats-Staats B, Woosley J, Morrell DS. Treatment of childhood kaposiform hemangioendothelioma with sirolimus. Pediatr Blood Cancer. 2010;55(7):1396–8.
12. Greene AK, Liu AS, Mulliken JB, Chalache K, Fishman SJ. Vascular anomalies in 5,621 patients: guidelines for referral. J Pediatr Surg. 2011;46(9):1784–9.
13. Mathes EF, Haggstrom AN, Dowd C, Hoffman WY, Frieden IJ. Clinical characteristics and management of vascular anomalies: findings of a multidisciplinary vascular anomalies clinic. Arch Dermatol. 2004;140(8):979–83.
14. Hassanein AH, Mulliken JB, Fishman SJ, Alomari AI, Zurakowski D, Greene AK. Venous malformation: risk of progression during childhood and adolescence. Ann Plast Surg. 2012;68(2):198–201.
15. Mazoyer E, Enjolras O, Bisdorff A, Perdu J, Wassef M, Drouet L. Coagulation disorders in patients with venous malformation of the limbs and trunk: a case series of 118 patients. Arch Dermatol. 2008;144(7):861–7.
16. Lee A, Driscoll D, Gloviczki P, Clay R, Shaughnessy W, Stans A. Evaluation and management of pain in patients with Klippel-Trenaunay syndrome: a review. Pediatrics. 2005;115(3):744–9.
17. Dompmartin A, Acher A, Thibon P, Tourbach S, Hermans C, Deneys V, Pocock B, Lequerrec A, Labbé D, Barrellier MT, Vanwijck R, Vikkula M, Boon LM. Association of localized intravascular coagulopathy with venous malformations. Arch Dermatol. 2008;144(7):873–7.
18. Rodríguez-Mañero M, Aguado L, Redondo P. Pulmonary arterial hypertension in patients with slow-flow vascular malformations. Arch Dermatol. 2010;146(12):1347–52.
19. Nguyen JT, Koerper MA, Hess CP, Dowd CF, Hoffman WY, Dickman M, Frieden IJ. Aspirin therapy in venous malformation: a retrospective cohort study of benefits, side effects, and patient experiences. Pediatr Dermatol. 2014;31(5):556–60.
20. Maguiness S, Koerper M, Frieden I. Relevance of D-dimer testing in patients with venous malformations. Arch Dermatol. 2009;145(11):1321–4.
21. Lance EI, Sreenivasan AK, Zabel TA, Kossoff EH, Comi AM. Aspirin use in Sturge-Weber syndrome: side effects and clinical outcomes. J Child Neurol. 2013;28(2):213–8.
22. Chiller KG, Passaro D, Frieden IJ. Hemangiomas of infancy: clinical characteristics, morphologic subtypes, and their relationship to race, ethnicity, and sex. Arch Dermatol. 2002;138(12):1567–76.
23. Suh KY, Frieden IJ. Infantile hemangiomas with minimal or arrested growth: a retrospective case series. Arch Dermatol. 2010;146(9):971–6.
24. Johnson EF, Smidt AC. Not just a diaper rash: LUMBAR syndrome. J Pediatr. 2014;164(1):208–9.
25. Stockman A, Boralevi F, Taïeb A, Léauté-Labrèze C. SACRAL syndrome: spinal dysraphism, anogenital, cutaneous, renal and urologic anomalies, associated with an angioma of lumbosacral localization. Dermatology. 2007;214(1):40–5.
26. Girard C, Bigorre M, Guillot B, Bessis D. PELVIS syndrome. Arch Dermatol. 2006;142(7):884–8.
27. Iacobas I, Burrows PE, Frieden IJ, Liang MG, Mulliken JB, Mancini AJ, Kramer D, Paller AS, Silverman R, Wagner AM, Metry DW. LUMBAR: association between cutaneous infantile hemangiomas of the lower body and regional congenital anomalies. J Pediatr. 2010;157(5):795–801.
28. Drolet BA, Chamlin SL, Garzon MC, Adams D, Baselga E, Haggstrom AN, Holland KE, Horii KA, Juern A, Lucky AW, Mancini AJ, McCuaig C, Metry DW, Morel KD, Newell BD,

Nopper AJ, Powell J, Frieden IJ. Prospective study of spinal anomalies in children with infantile hemangiomas of the lumbosacral skin. J Pediatr. 2010;157(5):789–94.

29. de Graaf M, Pasmans SG, van Drooge AM, Nievelstein RA, Gooskens RH, Raphael MF, Breugem CC. Associated anomalies and diagnostic approach in lumbosacral and perineal haemangiomas: case report and review of the literature. J Plast Reconstr Aesthet Surg. 2013;66(1):e26–8.

30. Willihnganz-Lawson K, Gordon J, Perkins J, Shnorhavorian M. Genitourinary and perineal vascular anomalies in children: a Seattle children's experience. J Pediatr Urol. 2015;11(4):227. e1–6.

31. Maguiness SM, Hoffman WY, McCalmont TH, Frieden IJ. Early white discoloration of infantile hemangioma: a sign of impending ulceration. Arch Dermatol. 2010;146(11):1235–9.

32. Maguiness SM, Frieden IJ. Management of difficult infantile haemangiomas. Arch Dis Child. 2012;97(3):266–71.

33. Thomas J, Kumar P, Kumar DD. Ulcerated infantile haemangioma of buttock successfully treated with topical timolol. J Cutan Aesthet Surg. 2013;6(3):168–9.

34. Michel JL, Patural H. Response to oral propranolol therapy for ulcerated hemangiomas in infancy. Arch Pediatr. 2009;16(12):1565–8.

35. Léauté-Labrèze C, Hoeger P, Mazereeuw-Hautier J, Guibaud L, Baselga E, Posiunas G, et al. A randomized, controlled trial of oral propranolol in infantile hemangioma. N Engl J Med. 2015;372(8):735–46.

36. Marqueling AL, Oza V, Frieden IJ, Puttgen KB. Propranolol and infantile hemangiomas four years later: a systematic review. Pediatr Dermatol. 2013;30(2):182–91.

37. Rogers M, Lam A, Fischer G. Sonographic findings in a series of rapidly involuting congenital hemangiomas (RICH). Pediatr Dermatol. 2002;19(1):5–11.

38. Enjolras O, Mulliken JB, Boon LM, Wassef M, Kozakewich HP, Burrows PE. Noninvoluting congenital hemangioma: a rare cutaneous vascular anomaly. Plast Reconstr Surg. 2001;107(7):1647–54.

39. Berenguer B, Mulliken JB, Enjolras O, Boon LM, Wassef M, Josset P, Burrows PE, Perez-Atayde AR, Kozakewich HP. Rapidly involuting congenital hemangioma: clinical and histopathologic features. Pediatr Dev Pathol. 2003;6(6):495–510.

40. Nasseri E, Piram M, McCuaig CC, Kokta V, Dubois J, Powell J. Partially involuting congenital hemangiomas: a report of 8 cases and review of the literature. J Am Acad Dermatol. 2014;70(1):75–9.

41. Boon LM, Enjolras O, Mulliken JB. Congenital hemangioma: evidence of accelerated involution. J Pediatr. 1996;128(3):329–35.

42. Maguiness S, Uihlein LC, Liang MG, Kozakewich H, Mulliken JB. Rapidly involuting congenital hemangioma with fetal involution. Pediatr Dermatol. 2015;32(3):321–6.

43. Elia D, Garel C, Enjolras O, Vermouneix L, Soupre V, Oury JF, Guibaud L. Prenatal imaging findings in rapidly involuting congenital hemangioma of the skull. Ultrasound Obstet Gynecol. 2008;31(5):572–5.

44. Fadell 2nd MF, Jones BV, Adams DM. Prenatal diagnosis and postnatal follow-up of rapidly involuting congenital hemangioma (RICH). Pediatr Radiol. 2011;41(8):1057–60.

45. Vildy S, Macher J, Abasq-Thomas C, Le Rouzic-Dartoy C, Brunelle F, Hamel-Teillac D, Duteille F, Perret C, Perrot P, Cassagnau E, Chauty-Frondas A, Aubert H, Barbarot S. Life-threatening hemorrhaging in neonatal ulcerated congenital hemangioma: two case reports. JAMA Dermatol. 2015;151(4):422–5.

46. Dickie B, Dasgupta R, Nair R, Alonso MH, Ryckman FC, Tiao GM, Adams DM, Azizkhan RG. Spectrum of hepatic hemangiomas: management and outcome. J Pediatr Surg. 2009;44(1):125–33.

47. Kulungowski AM, Alomari AI, Chawla A, Christison-Lagay ER, Fishman SJ. Lessons from a liver hemangioma registry: subtype classification. J Pediatr Surg. 2012;47(1):165–70.

48. Christison-Lagay ER, Burrows PE, Alomari A, Dubois J, Kozakewich HP, Lane TS, Paltiel HJ, Klement G, Mulliken JB, Fishman SJ. Hepatic hemangiomas: subtype classification and development of a clinical practice algorithm and registry. J Pediatr Surg. 2007;42(1):62–7.

49. Boon LM, Burrows PE, Paltiel HJ, Lund DP, Ezekowitz RA, Folkman J, Mulliken JB. Hepatic vascular anomalies in infancy: a twenty-seven-year experience. J Pediatr. 1996;129(3): 346–54.

50. Zenzen W, Perez-Atayde AR, Elisofon SA, Kim HB, Alomari AI. Hepatic failure in a rapidly involuting congenital hemangioma of the liver: failure of embolotherapy. Pediatr Radiol. 2009;39(10):1118–23.
51. North PE, Kahn T, Cordisco MR, Dadras SS, Detmar M, Frieden IJ. Multifocal lymphangio-endotheliomatosis with thrombocytopenia: a newly recognized clinicopathological entity. Arch Dermatol. 2004;140(5):599–606.
52. Prasad V, Fishman SJ, Mulliken JB, Fox VL, Liang MG, Klement G, Kieran MW, Burrows PE, Waltz DA, Powell J, Dubois J, Levy ML, Perez-Atayde AR, Kozakewich HP. Cutaneovisceral angiomatosis with thrombocytopenia. Pediatr Dev Pathol. 2005;8(4):407–19.
53. Marron M, Catrine K, North P, Browning MB, Kerschner JE, Noel R, Drolet BA, Kelly M. Expanding the phenotype of multifocal lymphangioendotheliomatosis with thrombocytopenia. Pediatr Blood Cancer. 2009;52(4):531–4.
54. Glick ZR, Frieden IJ, Garzon MC, Mully TW, Drolet BA. Diffuse neonatal hemangiomatosis: an evidence-based review of case reports in the literature. J Am Acad Dermatol. 2012;67(5): 898–903.
55. Nahm WK1, Moise S, Eichenfield LF, Paller AS, Nathanson L, Malicki DM, Friedlander SF. Venous malformations in blue rubber bleb nevus syndrome: variable onset of presentation. J Am Acad Dermatol. 2004 May;50(5 Suppl):S101-6.
56. Esparza EM, Deutsch G, Stanescu L, Weinberger E, Brandling-Bennett HA, Sidbury R. Multifocal lymphangioendotheliomatosis with thrombocytopenia: phenotypic variant and course with propranolol, corticosteroids, and aminocaproic acid. J Am Acad Dermatol. 2012;67(1):e62–4.
57. Kline RM, Buck LM. Bevacizumab treatment in multifocal lymphangioendotheliomatosis with thrombocytopenia. Pediatr Blood Cancer. 2009;52(4):534–6.
58. Droitcourt C, Boccara O, Fraitag S, Favrais G, Dupuy A, Maruani A. Multifocal lymphangio-endotheliomatosis with thrombocytopenia: clinical features and response to sirolimus. Pediatrics. 2015;136(2):e517–22.

Chapter 11
Abuse and Factitious Disorders

Kirsten Simonton and Kara N. Shah

Abstract Recognizing the cutaneous manifestations of child abuse, including physical and sexual abuse, is an important component of the medical evaluation in both the hospital-based and outpatient setting. Subtle clues on the skin examination may indicate the need for further evaluation, and the provider needs to be able to distinguish the features of injuries suspicious for non-accidental trauma from accidental skin injuries, medical conditions such as vasculitis, and skin signs of cultural practices such as cupping. Clinicians should also be able to recognize the signs of child neglect, in particular in high-risk situations or in cases where child abuse is also suspected. With regard to anogenital skin findings, sexual abuse should be considered when the lesions present indicate trauma. Finally, the possibility of self-induced skin lesions should always be considered when the history and/or examination is not consistent with a defined skin disorder.

Keywords Child physical abuse • Child sexual abuse • Child neglect • Ecchymoses • Thermal burn • Factitious disorder • Pathological skin picking

Case 11.1

History

A healthy 22-month-old male was admitted to the hospital by his primary care pediatrician due to a petechial rash and lethargy. He had been acting well at home until the day of admission, when his mother noted he was tired appearing, fussy, and had developed a rash on his face. He had no fevers, vomiting, cough, abdominal pain, or

K. Simonton, MD
Mayerson Center for Safe and Healthy Children, Cincinnati Children's Hospital,
3333 Burnet Avenue, MLC 3008, Cincinnati, OH, USA

K.N. Shah, MD, PhD (✉)
Division of Dermatology, Cincinnati Children's Hospital,
3333 Burnet Avenue, MLC 3004, Cincinnati, OH 45229, USA
e-mail: Kara.Shah@cchmc.org

© Springer International Publishing Switzerland 2016
M. Hogeling (ed.), *Case-Based Inpatient Pediatric Dermatology*,
DOI 10.1007/978-3-319-31569-0_11

pruritus. He was home with a babysitter during the day of admission while mother was at work. The babysitter did not report any trauma and stated that the rash developed after she gave him a piece of chocolate, and she thought he was having an allergic reaction. After giving him a dose of diphenhydramine with no change in symptoms or rash, the babysitter called his mother who came home early and brought him to the primary care pediatrician. Mother reports that he has met all appropriate developmental milestones.

Physical Exam

On physical examination, he is tired appearing and fussy. He is afebrile and mildly tachycardic. He has petechiae on his right ear, including the helix, antihelix, and posterior pinna, with small underlying ecchymoses (Fig. 11.1). Petechiae are also noted in the postauricular area without Battle's sign. A few scattered petechiae are seen just inferior to the right eye. The tympanic membranes are normal without perforation or hemotympanum. He has no apparent abdominal pain and no joint swelling or tenderness. Neurologic assessment is grossly nonfocal.

Fig. 11.1 On physical examination, grouped petechiae are noted on the pinna, helix, and antihelix

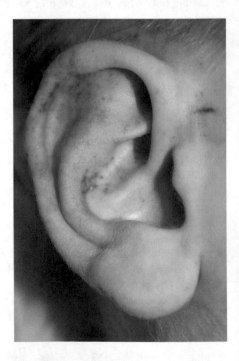

Laboratory Parameters

- White blood cells: 11.4 (6.0–17.0 K/mcL)
- Hemoglobin: 11.7 (11.5–13.5 g/dL)
- Platelet count: 215 (135–466 K/mcL)
- C-reactive protein: <0.21 (<+0.30 mg/dL)
- Activated partial thromboplastin time (APTT): 22.6 (21.7–31.6 s)
- Prothrombin time (PT): 11.5 (9.6–12.8 s)
- Urinalysis: normal

Questions

1. What is your differential diagnosis?
2. What further workup is appropriate for this patient?

Answer

The differential diagnosis of isolated petechiae with or without bruising includes inherited hematologic conditions including hemophilia and Von Willebrand (VW) disease, acquired platelet disorders including idiopathic thrombocytopenic purpura, other coagulopathies including vitamin K deficiency and disseminated intravascular coagulation, vasculitic disorders including Henoch–Schönlein purpura (HSP), and oncologic disorders including leukemia. Finally, accidental injury is a consideration when the mechanism described fits the location and extent of injuries and the developmental capabilities of the child.

In this patient, no history of trauma was provided, and laboratory evaluation including normal WBC, platelet count, APTT, and PT excludes the majority of the medical conditions on the differential. HSP is unlikely in this patient as the bruising does not involve dependent areas and he has no palpable purpura, abdominal pain, or joint swelling. The location of the petechiae and ecchymoses, normal hematologic evaluation, and lack of caregiver explanation for these clinical findings raise the suspicion for child abuse.

Skin injuries are the most common manifestations of child abuse, and bruising and petechiae are the most common skin injuries in children. Victims of child physical abuse often sustain trauma to the face and neck. While bruising to the head and face can occur from accidental injuries in a mobile child, certain bruising locations should prompt suspicion for abuse, including injuries of the auricle. The mnemonic "TEN 4" has been suggested to identify bruises that are concerning for abuse; these include T=torso, E=ear, N=neck, and 4=children less than or equal to 4 years of age and any bruising in infants under 4 months of age. Bruising of the anterior and posterior pinna is suggestive of pinching or pulling the ear, and bruising to the post-auricular area and antihelix in particular are uncommon locations for accidental injuries in young children [1].

The American Academy of Pediatrics (AAP) has recommended a thorough evaluation for bleeding disorders in children who have bruising or bleeding as part of their manifestation of possible child physical abuse. This includes a complete family history, past medical history and review of systems to identify the possibility of a bleeding disorder. Without a clear injury history or witnessed trauma, children with bruising should undergo initial hematologic testing including PT, APTT, VWF antigen, VWF activity, Factor VIII and Factor IX levels and a complete blood count including platelet count [2].

Young children who are suspected victims of child physical abuse should undergo evaluation for occult injuries. This includes laboratory evaluation for occult abdominal trauma including aspartate aminotransferase (AST) and alanine aminotransferase (ALT), and radiographic evaluation for occult skeletal trauma, which often consists of a skeletal survey [3]. A skeletal survey is a systematically performed series of 21 radiographic images that encompasses the entire skeleton. Data has suggested that a skeletal survey should be obtained in all children less than 24 months of age with concerns of physical abuse, and should be strongly considered in children as old as 36 months of age [4]. In children older than 36 months, a skeletal survey may have utility for children with significant developmental delays and those who are nonverbal. Neuroimaging should be obtained to evaluate for intracranial injury in young infants, in children with significant head or facial trauma, and in those with an abnormal neurologic examination. As our patient sustained injuries to the ear and face and was lethargic on admission, computed tomography (CT) of the head is indicated.

Treatment

Treatment of victims of child physical abuse will vary depending on the extent of injuries. Therefore, meticulous evaluation for occult trauma is essential, and will guide necessary interventions and follow-up. Children with isolated cutaneous injuries including bruising and petechiae often require no specific treatment apart from analgesics as needed. When there is uncertainty regarding whether a skin finding is a bruise rather than a congenital skin lesion or other dermatologic condition, repeat examinations can be helpful to follow the natural course of the lesions. Additionally, children who received an initial skeletal survey to evaluate for occult skeletal trauma should receive a follow-up skeletal survey 10–14 days later to assess for any healing fractures that may not have been visible on the initial study [1].

Definitive treatment for these children is removal from the abusive perpetrator and/or environment. Physicians are mandated reporters, and therefore are legally obligated to report any concerns for child abuse to their local child protective services or law enforcement agency. Furthermore, any siblings of the patient should be evaluated with a thorough physical examination and any indicated laboratory or radiologic evaluation to assess for the possibility of physical abuse. Children who have suffered abuse or neglect warrant close monitoring by caregivers and primary care physicians for behavioral problems, physical symptoms, and signs of psychological stress [1]. Trauma-focused therapies have demonstrated utility in children who exhibit symptoms related to past traumatic events.

Case 11.2

History

An 18-month-old female was admitted for observation after sustaining a right parietal skull fracture and small underlying subdural hematoma. Her parents state this occurred while she was climbing on playground equipment and fell onto concrete. They state that her head impacted the ground and no other injuries were sustained. On admission she was overall well appearing with a normal neurologic examination. Her mother noted that she has had a "bad diaper rash" for the past several days that has not been improving with use of a barrier cream. There is no history of diarrhea, urinary symptoms, or recent antibiotic use. Mother does note that they have been attempting to toilet train the patient recently, but she does continue to wear diapers during the day and night.

Physical Exam

On physical examination she is awake, alert, and mildly fussy. She has right-sided scalp edema without overlying lacerations or abrasions, and her neurologic examination is normal. She has ecchymoses to her mons pubis and petechiae on both labia majora with underlying ecchymoses (Fig. 11.2). Internal genitalia are normal including the labia minora and clitoral hood, and there is a crescentic hymen. There is no vaginal bleeding or discharge present. Perianal examination is normal.

Laboratory Parameters

- Hemoglobin: 11.9 (11.5–13.5 g/dL)
- Platelet count: 450 (135–466 K/mcL)
- Activated partial thromboplastin time (APTT): 21.9 (21.7–31.6 s)
- Prothrombin time (PT): 10.2 (9.6–12.8 s)
- Urinalysis: normal

Fig. 11.2 On physical examination, ecchymoses involving the mons pubis, scattered petechiae, and faint ecchymoses involving the labia majora are seen

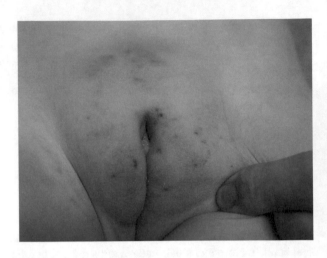

Questions

1. What diagnostic considerations are important in this patient?
2. What further workup is appropriate?

Answer

The physical findings noted in this patient—ecchymoses and petechiae of the external genitalia—indicate trauma concerning for child abuse. Accidental anogenital injury is relatively uncommon, particularly in children who wear diapers. Dermatitis is the most common vulvar condition seen in young children, and the most common dermatological condition seen in diapered children. Although the manifestations of diaper dermatitis can be extensive, including erythema, ulcerations, scaling and papules, evidence of ecchymoses or petechiae should alert the clinician to the possibility of trauma. As with other causes of bruising and petechiae, a hematologic evaluation is warranted to assess for coagulopathy, vasculitis, or other medical conditions predisposing to bruising. There is no evidence of a bleeding diathesis in this patient given her normal platelet count and coagulation studies. The indication of abusive injury to this child's external genitalia necessitates a complete evaluation for occult injury, including AST and ALT levels to assess for abdominal trauma, and a skeletal survey to assess for skeletal trauma. A more detailed history regarding the patient's head injury and a complete social assessment is also warranted.

Children who are victims of physical abuse may sustain injury to the genital or anal areas through a variety of mechanisms including burns, impact injury, biting, or penetrating trauma. Many abusive acts are in response to a child behavior that is negatively perceived by caregivers, and toilet training is a common trigger for physical abuse. However, it is important to recognize that children may sustain similar or identical injuries following sexual abuse. Therefore, although it can be difficult to distinguish whether the primary motivation of an injury is sexual in nature, an evaluation for further evidence of sexual abuse should be pursued [5].

When a history cannot be obtained from the patient due to developmental stage or other factors, the evaluation of possible sexual abuse includes a thorough physical examination and testing for evidence of sexual contact. Genital and anal examinations in children with concerns for sexual abuse should be performed by providers with adequate training and equipment to examine the patient, photo-document relevant findings, and make appropriate referrals. Sexually transmitted infections (STIs) occur infrequently following sexual abuse in prepubertal children. Therefore, the decision to test for STIs depends on a risk assessment for each individual child [6]. If evaluation for sexual abuse occurs in the acute setting, forensic evidence collection may also be indicated. As with any form of child maltreatment, physicians are mandated reporters and are legally obligated to report any suspicion of physical or sexual abuse to their local child protection services or law enforcement agency [7].

Treatment

Treatment of child abuse involves recognizing and anticipating the physical, emotional, and behavioral consequences that result from this trauma. Primary treatment beyond any necessary medical stabilization is removal of the child from the abusive perpetrator and/or environment. In cases of prepubertal child sexual abuse, testing for STIs may be appropriate if certain risk factors are present, including a history of genital or anal contact, perpetrator with known STI(s), or patient symptoms of an STI. When testing is performed, confirmatory testing of any positive results is often required in prepubertal children and in any case that involves the legal system. Prophylactic treatment for STIs in prepubertal children is generally not indicated except in significantly high-risk situations. Finally, children who have experienced child sexual abuse should be referred to a mental health professional with expertise in addressing childhood trauma [5, 7].

Case 11.3

History

A 4-year-old male with a history of asthma and mild atopic dermatitis is admitted for an acute asthma exacerbation. His mother reports that she "ran out of his asthma medications a while ago," and she has not requested refills from his primary care provider. He has been in the ED five times over the last year for asthma exacerbations and has required hospitalization three times for asthma. His father smokes cigarettes in the home, and his mother notes that smoke exposure is a frequent trigger for his asthma. His mother reports that his eczema is generally well controlled with emollients, but she has noticed new lesions on his left arm, and is now requesting a topical corticosteroid medication. His mother states she noticed the lesions 2 days ago when she returned home from work. He was home with his father and 2-year-old sister during the day, and his father stated that he hadn't noticed the lesions until the patient's mother pointed them out. She states that the lesions were never pustular or vesicular, there is no history of any bleeding or drainage, and the only change to the lesions over the past 2 days is that some have started to crust. He is noted to be delayed on his immunizations, and has received only one dose of the varicella vaccine.

Physical Exam

On physical examination he is receiving nebulized albuterol and is awake and alert in moderate respiratory distress. He is noted to be thin, with diffuse xerosis and numerous areas of dirt and debris on the skin, in his hair, and under the fingernails and toenails. His clothing is noted to be dirty and worn. Eczematous patches are noted in his antecubital and popliteal fossae bilaterally. Along the lateral aspect of the mid portion of his left upper extremity, there are five grouped superficial ulcers (Fig. 11.3). Each lesion is circular with sharply defined borders and measures 5–8 mm in diameter. The lesions have a punched-out appearance and are each surrounded by a ring of erythema. He has poor dentition.

Fig. 11.3 On physical examination, grouped, punched out circular superficial ulcers with surrounding erythema are noted involving the left arm

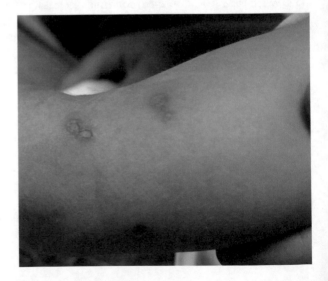

Laboratory Parameters

- White blood cells: 7.1 (5.0–19.5 K/mcL)
- Hemoglobin: 12.2 (11.5–13.5 g/dL)
- Platelet count: 350 (135–466 K/mcL)
- Bacterial culture (skin lesion): negative
- Fungal culture (skin lesion): negative

Questions

1. What is your differential diagnosis for this patient?
2. What is the appropriate treatment?

Answer

The differential diagnosis for grouped round skin lesions consistent with erosions and/or superficial ulcers is broad. Possible etiologies include infectious conditions, excoriations associated with pruritic disorders such as atopic dermatitis or contact dermatitis, unique cultural practices, and inflicted injury. A careful history, physical examination, and laboratory analysis help to differentiate these conditions. Diagnostic considerations may include impetigo; bacterial or fungal pyoderma; viral exanthems, including varicella and coxsackievirus; and certain folk remedies or alternative healing practices such as moxibustion, which may result in lesions with a similar appearance to inflicted burns. This practice consists of placing ground herbs often in conjunction with acupuncture needles and heat on the patient's skin, resulting in blistering and scarring at the site of impact. A careful history with specific questions regarding healing cultural practices will help uncover this diagnosis [8].

The lesions in this patient are consistent with inflicted cigarette burns. Accidental contact burns from a lit cigarette classically result in a single ill-defined oval or wedge-shaped lesion. They do not result in full-thickness skin injury due to the reflex withdrawal to pain of the affected body part. In contrast, inflicted cigarette burns have sharp round borders and usually appear in groups. Inflicted cigarette burns often produce a deep partial or full-thickness burn that is uniform in depth, and typically 5–10 mm in diameter depending on the size of the cigarette and the length of time it was applied to the skin. Lesions may blister, or may be dry and pale in appearance due to thermal coagulation of the involved tissue. These lesions heal gradually, often resulting in an atrophic scar with a hypopigmented center and hyperpigmented rim. Common locations for inflicted cigarette burns include the dorsum of hands and feet, face and limbs, although they can occur in any location.

Children with signs of physical abuse are also at risk for neglect, which includes physical neglect, emotional/psychological neglect, educational neglect, and medical neglect. Maltreatment by burning may be secondary to inflicted injury or supervisory neglect. Delayed presentation and lack of wound care prior to seeking medical attention are warning signs that a burn may be secondary to abuse or neglect. Burns resulting from abuse or neglect are also more likely to involve deeper tissue and require skin grafting [9]. Although this child's injury is consistent with intentional burning with a cigarette, he also manifests signs concerning for both physical and medical neglect including poor hygiene and attire, and a failure to provide appropriate care for his asthma and routine health maintenance.

Treatment

Children with inflicted burn injuries are at risk for other abusive injuries. In reports in the literature, intentional cigarette burns are frequently accompanied by other injuries, including blunt force injuries, evidence of sexual abuse, and occult fractures [10]. Current recommendations are to evaluate children with inflicted burns who are less than 24 months of age with a skeletal survey to assess for occult skeletal trauma [11]. In this 4-year-old patient, a full cutaneous and musculoskeletal examination is warranted to evaluate for any sign of further injuries.

When the diagnosis is uncertain, repeat examinations over the course of several days can help distinguish the expected progressive resolution of inflicted cigarette burns from the evolution of infectious conditions. Children who are verbal and of a certain cognitive and emotional maturity may be able to engage in a forensic interview to discuss how the lesions occurred.

Treatment of thermal burns is often supportive, and may involve analgesics, moisturizers, and topical antibiotics such as silver sulfadiazine to prevent and treat infections. Definitive treatment of child abuse involves removal of the child from the abusive perpetrator and/or environment, and anticipating the physical, emotional, and behavioral consequences that may result from the experienced trauma.

Neglect has the potential to adversely affect a child's psychosocial, cognitive, and emotional development, and has been shown to be a precursor for other forms of maltreatment, including physical abuse. Therefore, early detection of neglect has the potential to prevent further neglect as well as subsequent abuse. A multidisciplinary assessment is ideal in diagnosing neglect, and may include contact with the primary care provider, school, daycare setting, and other services that interact with the child. A social services assessment of the family including food insecurity, financial stressors, and living conditions in the home can significantly aid in the diagnosis of neglect. Just as in the diagnosis of neglect, treatment is most effective when done as a multidisciplinary effort, and involves addressing both the physical and psychosocial aspects of neglect. A treatment team may include the primary care physician, child behavioral specialists, social workers, home visitors, parent and child educators, and mental health professionals. While a report to child protective services is mandatory in cases of suspected neglect, a determination of removal from the home is made on an individual basis, and in some cases, services may be provided to the family while the child remains in the home. Appropriate reporting and service referral can help ameliorate the significant risks associated with maltreatment secondary to neglect.

Case 11.4

History

A 16-year-old girl with a history of anxiety is admitted with a several month history of a chronic, asymptomatic rash on her chest and a 3-week history of right axillary lymphadenitis. There is no history of fever or arthralgias. Prior outpatient evaluation of the rash was remarkable for methicillin-resistant *Staphylococcus aureus* (MRSA) on superficial bacterial culture; prior treatment with both topical mupirocin ointment and oral trimethoprim-sulfamethoxazole as prescribed by her primary care provider were of limited efficacy and the rash has persisted. She denies symptoms such as pain or pruritus, and denies picking or scratching. She is unable to provide a history of the eruption. She has a history of anxiety and her grandfather has been recently diagnosed with leukemia. Current medications include fluoxetine and clindamycin.

Physical Exam

She was well appearing and afebrile on examination. Involving the superior portion of the breasts, there are several scattered, discrete 5–10 mm erythematous crusted round erosions and a few superficial ulcers admixed with resolving erythematous slightly atrophic macules (Fig. 11.4). There is a 3 cm tender, non-fluctuant minimally erythematous subcutaneous nodule in the right axillae.

Laboratory Parameters

- WBC: 7.1 (4.5–13.5 K/mcL)
- Erythrocyte sedimentation rate: 8 (<20 mm/h)
- C-reactive protein: 0.3 (<1.0 mg/dL)
- HSV PCR (skin lesion): negative
- VSV PCR (skin lesion): negative
- Bacterial culture (skin lesion): negative
- Skin biopsy: ulceration of the epidermis with serosanguinous crust, mild mixed inflammation of the superficial dermis

Fig. 11.4 On physical examination, there are scattered erythematous crusted round erosions, superficial ulcers, and resolving erythematous slightly atrophic macules on the upper chest

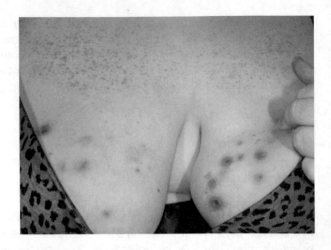

Questions

1. What is your differential diagnosis for these clinical findings?
2. What diagnostic clues can facilitate arriving at the correct diagnosis?

Answer

Diagnostic considerations for localized cutaneous erosions and superficial ulcers may include infection (more commonly bacterial (e.g., Staphylococcal, Streptococcal ecthyma, or other presentation) or viral (e.g., herpes simplex virus, varicella zoster virus, or enterovirus), arthropod infestation (e.g., scabies, bedbugs), vasculitis, inflammatory dermatoses such as pityriasis lichenoides et varioliformis acuta and some presentations of collagen vascular disease, and autoimmune bullous disease (e.g., dermatitis herpetiformis). The differential diagnosis also includes a self-inflicted skin lesion (SISL), historically referred to as dermatitis artefacta. On the basis of the history of anxiety, inability of the patient to provide a concrete history for the cutaneous manifestations, clinical features, negative diagnostic testing, and skin biopsy supportive of induced trauma, a diagnosis of a factitious skin disorder was rendered.

SISLs in children can present a significant diagnostic dilemma, and they are often not considered in the differential diagnosis of a cutaneous eruption. The European Society for Dermatology and Psychiatry defines SISL as "any skin lesion actively and directly produced by the patient on his/her skin, mucosa or integument that is not better explained as a consequence of another physical or mental disorder" [12]. These clinical behaviors are the result of a maladaptive response to one or more internal psychological stressors. If the presentation involves the deliberate invocation of the cutaneous manifestations for secondary gain (e.g., avoidance of school or an abusive caregiver), and the behavior is denied, malingering is diagnosed; if there is no secondary gain but the behavior is denied, a factitious disorder is diagnosed. If the patient readily admits to inducing the skin lesions, a compulsive or impulsive skin picking/skin damaging syndrome is diagnosed. The presence of an associated mental health disorder such as depression or anxiety is common, and in adults, SISL appears more commonly in women. Examples of common SISL in children and adolescents include trichotillomania, acne excorièe, and factitial purpura [13, 14].

Clues to the diagnosis may include a vague or "hollow" history; skin lesions that are bizarre or oddly geometric; involvement of readily accessible areas such as the anterior extremities, face, chest, and upper back; lesions that do not conform in distribution and morphology to any known dermatologic disease or condition; and the appearance that the patient is indifferent to the cutaneous manifestations.

Evaluation may necessitate performing a skin biopsy or other diagnostic testing to exclude other diagnostic considerations and to convince the patient and caregivers of the correct diagnosis. The diagnosis is one of exclusion, although it is often suspected clinically.

Treatment

Perhaps the most critical component of treatment of self-induced skin lesions in children is the establishment of a trusting and therapeutic physician–patient–caregiver relationship [13]. Patients and caregivers need to feel supported in a nonjudgmental manner, which can be a challenge for the provider as many patients and caregivers are very resistant to the concept of a self-induced process and are determined to seek an alternative diagnosis. As such, it may take several encounters with the patient and caregiver for the provider to establish the degree of rapport needed to be able to introduce the idea of a SISL while minimizing the risk of alienating the patient and caregiver. Excluding a diagnosis of a primary skin disease or other primary disorder with cutaneous manifestations is also an important component of management.

Involving a behavioral health provider such a pediatric clinical psychologist early in the process can be helpful, though the initial referral may seek to address concerns such as coping or stress [13]. Cognitive behavioral therapy and other forms of psychotherapy are an important component of treatment. Psychopharmacologic intervention may be considered for patients with associated mental health comorbidities that cannot be adequately addressed with psychotherapy alone, and should be made with the assistance of a psychiatrist or other mental health provider with expertise in this area. Medical therapy consists predominantly of wound care, if appropriate, including management of any secondary infection.

The prognosis for SISL in children appears more favorable than that in adults, and younger children appear to have the best prognosis, although the course may be protracted over several years and characterized by chronicity and intermittent recurrences.

References

1. Christian CW, Committee on Child A, Neglect AAoP. The evaluation of suspected child physical abuse. Pediatrics. 2015;135(5):e1337–54.
2. Anderst JD, Carpenter SL, Abshire TC, Section on HO, Committee on Child A, Neglect of the American Academy of P. Evaluation for bleeding disorders in suspected child abuse. Pediatrics. 2013;131(4):e1314–22.
3. Harper NS, Feldman KW, Sugar NF, Anderst JD, Lindberg DM, Examining Siblings To Recognize Abuse I. Additional injuries in young infants with concern for abuse and apparently isolated bruises. J Pediatr. 2014;165(2):383–8 e1.
4. Lindberg DM, Berger RP, Reynolds MS, Alwan RM, Harper NS, Examining Siblings To Recognize Abuse I. Yield of skeletal survey by age in children referred to abuse specialists. J Pediatr. 2014;164(6):1268–73 e1.
5. Kellogg N, American Academy of Pediatrics Committee on Child A, Neglect. The evaluation of sexual abuse in children. Pediatrics. 2005;116(2):506–12.
6. Girardet RG, Lahoti S, Howard LA, Fajman NN, Sawyer MK, Driebe EM, et al. Epidemiology of sexually transmitted infections in suspected child victims of sexual assault. Pediatrics. 2009;124(1):79–86.
7. Jenny C, Crawford-Jakubiak JE, Committee on Child A, Neglect, American Academy of P. The evaluation of children in the primary care setting when sexual abuse is suspected. Pediatrics. 2013;132(2):e558–67.
8. Faller-Marquardt M, Pollak S, Schmidt U. Cigarette burns in forensic medicine. Forensic Sci Int. 2008;176(2–3):200–8.
9. Chester DL, Jose RM, Aldlyami E, King H, Moiemen NS. Non-accidental burns in children—are we neglecting neglect? Burns. 2006;32(2):222–8.
10. Kemp AM, Maguire SA, Lumb RC, Harris SM, Mann MK. Contact, cigarette and flame burns in physical abuse: a systematic review. Child Abuse Rev. 2014;23(1):35–47.
11. Degraw M, Hicks RA, Lindberg D, Using Liver Transaminases to Recognize Abuse Study I. Incidence of fractures among children with burns with concern regarding abuse. Pediatrics. 2010;125(2):e295–9.
12. Gieler U, Consoli SG, Tomas-Aragones L, Linder DM, Jemec GB, Poot F, et al. Self-inflicted lesions in dermatology: terminology and classification—a position paper from the European Society for Dermatology and Psychiatry (ESDaP). Acta Derm Venereol. 2013;93(1):4–12.
13. Shah KN, Fried RG. Factitial dermatoses in children. Curr Opin Pediatr. 2006;18(4):403–9.
14. Chiriac A, Brzezinski P, Pinteala T, Chiriac AE, Foia L. Common psychocutaneous disorders in children. Neuropsychiatr Dis Treat. 2015;11:333–7.

Chapter 12
Bullous Disorders of Childhood

Marion E. Tamesis and Kimberly D. Morel

Abstract Bullous diseases, both inherited and autoimmune, may be encountered on the inpatient consultation service. Neonates may be born with blisters and it is important to be aware of first and foremost the importance of ruling out an infectious process. The family history and morphology of the lesions may provide important clues to the diagnosis. Once infection has been ruled out, in cases without a family history of bullous disease, the autosomal recessive forms of genetically inherited blistering disease such as epidermolysis bullosa although rare, are more common than the autoimmune bullous disease in neonates. Acquired forms of blistering in the category of autoimmune remain rare, but become more common as children mature. Sudden presentations of large acral blisters in infants should prompt consideration of infantile bullous pemphigoid after hand-foot-mouth disease or other infection is ruled out. Linear IgA bullous disease, also known as chronic bullous disease of childhood, is often initially mistaken for impetigo and although may be superinfected and partially respond to oral antibiotics, the diagnosis may only become clear with the clinical course or the astute clinician recognizing and initiating a workup for the condition. Regardless of the cause of the blisters, careful wound care with non-adherent dressings and monitoring for signs or symptoms of superinfection must be performed.

Keywords Autoimmune bullous disease • Bullous • Chronic bullous disease of childhood • Direct immunofluorescence • Epidermolysis bullosa • Infantile bullous pemphigoid • Linear IgA bullous disease (LAD) of childhood

M.E. Tamesis, MD
Department of Dermatology, New York Presbyterian Hospital, Columbia University Medical Center, 161 Fort Washington Avenue, Herbert Irving Pavilion, 12th Floor, Room 1218, New York, NY 10032, USA
e-mail: mt3008@cumc.columbia.edu

K.D. Morel, MD, FAAD, FAAP (✉)
Department of Dermatology and Pediatrics, Morgan Stanley Children's Hospital of New York-Presbyterian/Columbia University, 161 Fort Washington Avenue, 12th Floor, New York, NY 10032, USA
e-mail: km208@cumc.columbia.edu; km208@columbia.edu

© Springer International Publishing Switzerland 2016
M. Hogeling (ed.), *Case-Based Inpatient Pediatric Dermatology*,
DOI 10.1007/978-3-319-31569-0_12

Case 12.1

History

A 1-day-old full term baby girl is noted to have absent skin on her lower extremities at birth. Her nurses have noted blisters and erosions at sites where tape and monitor leads were placed after delivery. The neonatology team has initiated a rule out sepsis workup and performed initial bacterial and viral cultures on the erosions. Dermatology is consulted for further evaluation.

Physical Examination (Fig. 12.1)

On physical examination, linear erosions were present over her shins and dorsal feet bilaterally. Flaccid bullae were present on her heels. Several vesicles were present on her abdomen and erosions were present at prior cardiac monitor adhesive sites. Nails were absent on the affected toenails.

Laboratory Parameters

- White blood cell count: 12 $(8–30 \times 10(9) \, L^{-1})$

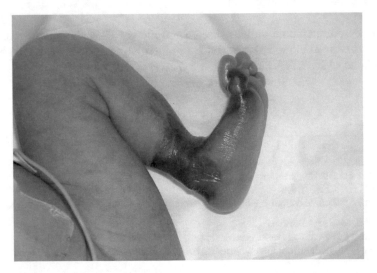

Fig. 12.1 Congenital localized absence of skin of the distal lower extremity and medial foot. Small first toe with absent nail

- Hemoglobin: 16.5 (13.5–19.5 g%)
- Hematocrit: 49.5 (42–60 %)
- Platelet count: 290 (165–415 × 10(9) L^{-1})
- HSV and VZV DFA: negative
- Gram stain or wound erosion: no polys, no organisms.
- Wound culture: negative to date.
- HSV: herpes simplex virus; VZV: varicella zoster virus; DFA: direct fluorescence antibody.

Questions

1. What is your differential diagnosis?
2. What investigations would you order/how would you approach this patient?
3. What are your typical histopathological findings?
4. What treatment would you consider?

Answers

Differential Diagnosis

Blistering and erosions in the newborn period may be seen in a variety of medical conditions. The clue in this patient that points towards a diagnosis of epidermolysis bullosa is the linear aplasia cutis on the extremities, also referred to as congenital localized absence of skin, in association with skin fragility. The linear aplasia cutis is not present in all patients with EB but when noted should prompt evaluation for this condition. It is important to note that it is not possible to determine subtype of EB (namely Dystrophic EB, Junctional EB, EB Simplex, Kindler syndrome) nor predict outcomes based on the clinical phenotype in the neonatal period.

As in older children, it is important to first rule out infectious causes which can be life-threatening if not promptly treated. Linear erosions and blisters, even infections such as HSV and VZV, can mimic EB [1, 2]. Infectious causes that must be considered include bacterial infections such as staph scalded skin syndrome (SSSS), Group B streptococcus, and pseudomonas and other infections such as herpes simplex virus, varicella, and syphilis. More often in seriously ill and premature infants, deep fungal infections such as Aspergillus have also been reported to present with vesicles (see below).

The differential diagnosis also includes autoimmune causes of blistering which in the neonatal period are even rarer than genetically inherited causes such as epidermolysis bullosa, especially when there is no maternal history of autoantibodies. Autoimmune blistering disorders may occur in the neonatal period due to transplacental transmission of maternal antibodies. A maternal history is helpful, although absence of maternal history of disease does not rule out the disease as rare cases have been reported from an asymptomatic mother. Neonatal lupus generally presents with annular lesions, but may present with widespread erosions in the neonatal period. Pemphigus vulgaris and pemphigus foliaceous may also present in this manner. Rare cases of Epidermolysis Bullosa Acquisita (EBA) and chronic bullous disease of childhood have been reported. Bullous pemphigoid has been reported in infants, although onset is most often after 2 months of age.

A number of other noninfectious causes can present with newborn blisters (see below). Many are exceedingly rare. An example is cutaneous mast cell disease. The most common presentation is that of a single or several lesions, mastocytomas, which urticate when rubbed (positive Darier's sign) and secondary blistering may occur. Infants with widespread cutaneous lesions may have more severe generalized blistering.

Differential Diagnosis of the Neonate with Blisters
Epidermolysis bullosa
Staphylococcal scalded skin syndrome
Herpes simplex virus
Other infections: syphilis, GBS, pseudomonas, aspergillus, varicella, other

    CMV, EBV, mycoplasma, Chikungunya virus

Autoimmune:

    Transplacental maternal antibodies: pemphigus vulgaris, foliaceous, EBA
    Chronic bullous disease of childhood—case report
    Bullous pemphigoid (usually after 2 mo)
    Neonatal lupus erythematosus—can present with widespread erosions

Epidermolytic hyperkeratosis/epidermolytic ichthyosis
Kindler syndrome
Scabies
Diffuse cutaneous mastocytosis
Congenital erosive and vesicular dermatosis
Congenital self-healing reticulohistiocytosis
Toxic epidermal necrolysis—due to intrauterine graft versus host disease or neonatal gram negative sepsis
Porphyrias
Protein C and S deficiency (hemorrhagic bullae)
Incontinentia pigmenti
Sucking blisters

The Approach to the Newborn with Blisters

The history of the newborn should of course focus on the perinatal history and family history. Questions should be sought regarding maternal history of herpes simplex virus, syphilis, or other bacterial infections. Maternal laboratory studies should be reviewed. Family history should be obtained including any history of skin blistering or skin fragility including transient blistering in the newborn period. Nail dystrophy or dental abnormalities in the family should be asked about as it can also be a manifestation of certain genetically inherited conditions associated with newborn skin fragility. Maternal history of autoimmune disease is especially important to inquire about as maternal transmission of transplacental antibodies can affect the newborn for several months after delivery. On physical examination, the morphology and location of the lesions may provide clues to the diagnosis. Infections such as HSV may present with clusters of vesicles on an erythematous base, on scalp and presenting parts such as shoulders more often than other sites. Erosions even without blisters especially in preterm infants may be a presenting sign of cutaneous bacterial, viral, or fungal infections. Linear vesicles can be a clue to other genetically inherited disorders such as incontinentia pigmenti. However, do not become too confident in your clinical assessment, HSV has been reported to mimic the presentation of noninfectious bullous disorders and vice versa. If clinical suspicion for infection is high, treatment should be initiated promptly without waiting for results and should be continued regardless of preliminary results [3].

Typical Histological Findings

When epidermolysis bullosa is suspected, a biopsy of a freshly induced blister is the most helpful tool to try to define the subtype of EB in the short term [4, 5]. The method of inducing a blister can be done by twisting with a gloved finger or clean pencil eraser [6]. Twisting must be performed gently at first as skin separation may form with the mildest shearing force in severe cases. Progressively stronger twists are performed until at least erythema develops. If a blister is not immediately visualized, giving the site time to accumulate fluid is the next step. A punch biopsy is performed to include an edge of intact skin so that the blister roof does not completely separate from the sample. The level of split and absent or abnormal protein staining including Collagen VII, Type XVII collagen, laminin 332, and integrins can be assessed by Direct Immunofluorescence (DIF) testing at select laboratories that perform this testing [Beutner Laboratories or Stanford University Dermatopathology]. The results can help determine subtype of epidermolysis bullosa. Inability to induce a blister does not rule out EB but could indicate a higher threshold for blistering with a milder phenotype or a mosaic form of the disease. Also note, performing a biopsy on a previously formed blister will not yield diagnostic DIF results due to the inflammation that occurs, even when a blister may appear to have been of recent onset. A fresh blister must be induced as a previously present blister will have inflammation which will interfere with the test results.

Routine histology is not generally helpful in determining EB subtype but can help in certain other conditions. (Example: in a patient with erythematous tender skin and a positive Nikolsky's sign, separation at the level of the stratum granulosum is supportive of a diagnosis of SSSS or spongiosis with eosinophils as may be seen in the linear plaques of Incontinentia Pigmenti.) There is no role for indirect immunofluorescence in the diagnosis of inherited epidermolysis bullosa. Advances in genetic testing have made it possible to test whole exome sequencing for mutations associated with known subtypes of EB [7].

Treatment

Once the diagnosis of EB has been established and there are no signs or symptoms of infection, treatment is supportive and geared towards careful wound care with non-adherent dressings [8]. There is currently no available cure for this life-altering condition. Supportive care is provided with topical antibiotics and non-adherent dressing to wounds when present. Careful consideration of topical ointments to apply must be undertaken. Systemic absorption of topically applied substances occurs in neonatal skin, and erosions are even more likely to be associated with increased systemic absorption of topically applied substances. For example, topical neomycin should be avoided, given the risk of ototoxicity with systemic absorption [9]. Multiple specialists are frequently required in the interdisciplinary care of this disease. Nursing care and parent education in the careful and often time-consuming care are essential from early on. Regardless of the cause of the lesions, the body surface area of involvement of blisters and erosions must be noted so that the increased fluid and nutritional requirements can be calculated. Gastroenterologists and nutritionists are helpful in managing the increased caloric and nutritional requirements to stay ahead of the known risk of failure to thrive. Use of a Habermann nipple, pre-moistened before feeds, may be helpful. Consultation of a feeding specialist is often recommended from early on. Pain management is also important and must be balanced with avoiding over sedation which may interfere with feeding and maintaining caloric and nutritional requirements. Adhesives should not come in contact directly with the skin lest they cause more blisters and erosions and so securing lines may be difficult. Pediatric Dermatologists are often called upon to relay information regarding care of fragile skin. The Dystrophic Epidermolysis Bullosa Research Association (DEBRA.org) is a helpful resource for patient care questions and families affected by this condition. Genetics and genetic counseling are an important resource for the option of genetic diagnosis of the known EB subtypes. Options for research protocols underway can be searched on clinicaltrials.gov.

Case 12.2

History

An 8-year-old male presents for evaluation with a 2-month history of intermittent vesicular and erythematous annular eruption usually affecting his perioral region, trunk, and extremities. The current rash has been present for the past few days, this time with extensive yellow crusted plaques and vesicles around his mouth, trunk, and upper and lower extremities. He is admitted for IV antibiotic administration with concern for widespread impetigo. He denies any fever, throat pain, dysuria, or other systemic complaints. He denies intake of any medications. Dermatology is consulted for further evaluation.

Physical Exam (Fig. 12.2)

On physical examination, vesicles, erosions, and erythematous, annular patches and plaques with arcuate and serpiginous borders are present. One erosion on his cheek is rimmed by an annular rosette of tense vesicles. He has lesions periorally, on the lower abdomen, arms, and upper thighs. Nikolsky sign is negative. He has mild conjunctival injection but no other ocular findings. No other mucosal lesions are present.

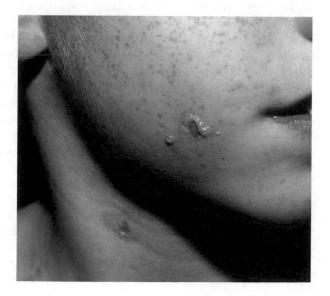

Fig 12.2 Physical examination showed grouped vesicles and bullae in an annular shape similar to a "string of pearls." From Mintz EM, Morel KD. Chronic bullous disease of childhood. Derm Clinics 2011;29(3):459–462. Reprinted with permission from Elsevier Limited

Laboratory Parameters

- White blood count: 8.0 (4.0–10.5 K/μL)
- Hemoglobin: 13.2 (11.5–13.5 g/dL)
- Hematocrit: 39.1 (34.0–40.0 %)
- Platelet count: 311 ($165–415 \times 10^9$ L^{-1})
- HSV and VZV DFA: negative
- Tzanck smear: negative
- Gram stain of blister fluid: no organisms
- Wound culture: negative to date
- Skin biopsy of perilesional skin revealed papillary dermal edema, a subepidermal bullae with a mixed infiltrate of mononuclear cells and neutrophils. DIF showed linear deposits of IgA, C3, and IgG at the basement membrane zone.

Questions

1. What is your differential diagnosis?
2. What investigations would you order?
3. What are the typical histopathologic findings?
4. What treatment would you consider?

Answers

Differential Diagnosis

Based on the patient's history, physical examination, and biopsy results, this patient has linear IgA bullous dermatosis (LABD) of childhood also known as chronic bullous disease of childhood. This entity was previously thought to be a childhood form of dermatitis herpetiformis then later reclassified as bullous pemphigoid of childhood. Currently, this condition is widely recognized to be a distinct autoimmune mucocutaneous disorder due to IgA antibodies against the basement membrane of the skin and mucous membranes causing a subepidermal blister and characteristic immunofluorescent findings [10]. LABD of childhood usually occurs between 6 months and 6 years of age. An adult form can be seen after puberty, generally in the seventh decade of life. Some sources report a slight female predominance; however, more recent data suggest a heterogeneous sex ratio worldwide. Although most children have self-limited disease that resolves within 3–6 years, many require systemic therapy during the active phase to control blistering. Evaluation for the possibility of mucosal involvement early in the course of the disease is important as ocular involvement with scarring can lead to blindness and upper airway involvement leading to stenosis and breathing impairment [10].

Typical exam findings include tense, clear, or hemorrhagic vesicles and bullae grouped in an annular arrangement similar to a "string of pearls." These may be seen on normal skin or on an erythematous or urticarial base and are commonly found in the lower abdomen, anogenital region, and lower extremities. A few patients may have a sudden onset of a rash with fever and constitutional symptoms [10, 11]. LABD of childhood may be idiopathic or caused by an identifiable trigger. Precipitating factors that have been reported include medications, systemic illness, ultraviolet light exposure, and other traumatic events. The pathogenesis behind the autoimmune response triggered by the above factors still remains unknown. Many antigens have been identified as being involved in the pathophysiology of LABD and the targeted antigens are located in the basement membrane zone of the stratified squamous epithelium of the skin and mucous membranes [10–12].

The differential diagnosis of bullous eruptions in childhood is broad. Initially, it is most important to rule out an infectious process such as impetigo, herpes simplex virus, or varicella zoster virus. After infection has been ruled out or for long-standing symptoms, the possibility of autoimmune blistering diseases must be considered. The morphology of the rash should also point towards certain autoimmune disease even early in the presentation. Autoimmune diseases in childhood also include childhood bullous pemphigoid, childhood dermatitis herpetiformis, and EBA. Childhood bullous pemphigoid is much less common in children versus adults and usually presents with symmetrical, ungrouped blisters of variable size, located primarily on flexural surfaces of the trunk and extremities [13, 14]. The childhood form of dermatitis herpetiformis commonly presents as a burning or pruritic papulovesicular eruption distributed symmetrically especially on the scalp, buttocks, and extensor surfaces of the extremities [12]. EBA is characterized by skin fragility, predilection for the hands, feet, elbows, and knees, and mucosal/extracutaneous involvement [12]. A non-scarring inflammatory form of EBA may affect children, whereas healing with atrophy, milia, scars, and dyspigmentation is seen more often in the adult non-inflammatory form of this condition [15]. Clues to other bullous disorders in the differential diagnosis include the linear nature of poison ivy dermatitis which may present with intensely pruritic papules, vesicles, and bullae, the non-migratory annular to bullous rash that appear in the same body site in a fixed drug eruption, the sharply demarcated borders and geometric shapes in contact dermatitis, and the red to brown patches that urticate and blister with rubbing in urticaria pigmentosa (cutaneous mastocytosis).

Serious bullous disorders such as Stevens–Johnson syndrome (SJS), Sweet's syndrome, and bullous Henoch–Schönlein Purpura (HSP) should also be considered. SJS more often presents with mucosal lesions and atypical target and purpuric macules that rapidly progress to large bullae and epidermal necrosis in an ill-appearing child [16]. Sweet's syndrome commonly involves the hands and other acral sites with dark red, thick, well-demarcated plaques that may appear to have vesicles [17]. HSP manifests as palpable purpura that may form hemorrhagic bullae and necrotic ulcers in dependent sites such as the buttocks and extensor extremities.

Histopathologic Findings

A skin biopsy may demonstrate a subepidermal vesicle or bullae with a neutrophilic dermal infiltrate. DIF of perilesional skin shows linear deposits of IgA at the basement membrane zone. The main target antigen is BP 180 (or collagen XVII), a key structural component of the dermoepidermal junction adhesion complex [11]. In about 80 % of patients, indirect immunofluorescence demonstrates circulating IgA antibodies, as well as C3 and IgG [10].

Treatment

LABD of childhood is generally self-limited and usually resolves by puberty. Antibiotics with reported success in treating LABD of childhood, especially as an initial or temporizing agent, include erythromycin, dicloxacillin, and oxacillin [18, 19]. Drug of choice for long-term systemic therapy is dapsone. Dapsone is usually started at a low dose (<0.5 mg/kg) and slowly titrated until few to no lesions are observed (usually at 2 mg/kg). Alternatively, sulfapyridine may be given at 150 mg/kg/day. Adverse effects of dapsone and related medications include hemolysis, methemoglobinemia, agranulocytosis, peripheral neuropathy, hepatitis, GI upset, cutaneous hypersensitivity reactions, and dapsone hypersensitivity syndrome. Prior to initiating therapy with dapsone or the alternative sulfapyridine, patients should be screened for G6PD deficiency. CBC, LFTs, and renal function tests should be monitored carefully while on either medication [20, 21]. Prednisone may be added temporarily to control severe disease. The long-term nature of this condition makes systemic steroids a less ideal choice for maintenance therapy, given its side effects with prolonged use. Alternative therapies for those in whom dapsone or sulfapyridine is contraindicated include colchicine and nicotinamide [20].

Conclusion

Chronic bullous disease of childhood or LABD of childhood is an autoimmune disorder due to IgA antibodies against the basement membrane of the skin and mucous membranes. Clinically, this presents as tense vesicles and bullae grouped in a "string of pearls" configuration on the lower abdomen, groin, and lower extremities. Histologically, this causes a subepidermal blister on H&E and characteristic linear deposits of IgA at the basement membrane zone on direct immunofluorescence of perilesional skin. This is generally self-limited but severe cases have been successfully treated with dapsone.

Case 12.3

History

A 6-month-old female who presented with a 5-day history of a bullous eruption that first appeared as urticarial plaques on her hands and feet then spread to her trunk. She was afebrile but was irritable and had decreased oral intake. She was subsequently admitted for failure to tolerate PO and dermatology was consulted for evaluation of the eruption. She was seen by her pediatrician 1 week prior to the onset of her symptoms for her well-baby visit. At that visit, she received her first dose of diphtheria, tetanus, acellular pertussis (DtaP), Haemophilus influenza B, inactivated polio virus, and pneumococcal conjugate vaccines. She had no prior history of a similar eruption and there is no family history of any chronic skin conditions. There was no intake of new medications or use new products. There was no recent travel or ill contacts. There was no family history of autoimmune disease or blistering disorders.

Physical Exam (Fig. 12.3)

Laboratory Parameters

- White blood count: 8.0 (5.0–17.5 K/μL)
- Hemoglobin: 11.4 (11.3–14.1 g/dL)
- Hematocrit: 34.2 (31.0–41.0 %)

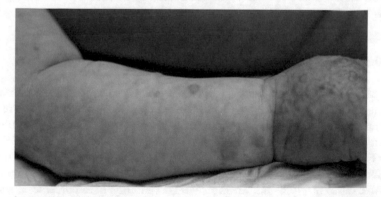

Fig 12.3 Physical examination revealed tense vesicles with surrounding erythema on the hands. Tense bullae were present on the soles and urticarial plaques were present on the trunk. From Weitz NA, Mintz EM, Morel KD. Autoimmune Bullous Diseases of Childhood. In: Severe Skin Diseases in Children beyond Topical Therapy. Ed. Tom W. Springer 2014. Reprinted with permission from Springer

- Platelet count: 250 $(150–350 \times 10^9 \text{ L}^{-1})$
- Eosinophils: 7 % (2–6%)
- HSV and VZV DFA: negative
- Tzanck smear: negative for multinucleated giant cells
- Gram stain of blister fluid: no organisms
- Wound culture: negative to date
- Skin biopsy of lesional skin revealed a subepidermal bulla with a perivascular eosinophilic and lymphocytic infiltrate
- DIF on non-lesional skin revealed linear deposits of IgG and C3 at the basement membrane zone

Questions

1. What is your differential diagnosis?
2. What investigations would you order?
3. What are the typical histopathologic findings?
4. What treatment would you consider?

Answers

Differential Diagnosis

As discussed in "Case 12.2" section, the differential diagnosis of bullous eruptions in infants and children is broad. First and foremost, especially in younger children, infection must be ruled out. Infections in infants may present with bullae, especially bullous impetigo or SSSS.

Investigations

Appropriate initial tests to perform include a Tzanck smear to evaluate for multi-nucleated giant cells, viral direct fluorescent antibody or polymerase chain reaction and viral cultures to evaluate for viral illness, a gram stain and bacterial culture to evaluate for impetigo. Note that in certain bacterial infections, especially SSSS, bullae may be secondary to a toxin at a site other than skin and so additional sources of infection other than skin should be considered. SSSS usually presents differently as an abrupt onset of erythema, fever, malaise, irritability, skin tenderness, and erythema, followed by formation of large fluid filled bullae and diffuse epidermal desquamation [22, 23].

SJS should be considered especially in children with mucosal lesions. However, patients with SJS tend to be ill-appearing, with widespread blisters and erythematous or purpuric macules, and have a relatively more acute and rapidly progressive course. Similarly, erythema multiforme may present as a symmetric cutaneous eruption that evolve within days to the classic target to bullous lesions with minimal or no mucosal involvement [16]. Linear IgA dermatosis frequently appears with the string of pearls configuration of bullae on the lower abdomen, anogenital region, and lower extremities [10]. These conditions may be differentiated by doing an H&E, direct and indirect immunofluorescent studies.

Other bullous disorders to consider include contact dermatitis which appear as well-demarcated, geometric, or odd-shaped vesiculobullous eruption, bullous arthropod reaction which is characterized by pruritic local erythema and edema with or without a central punctum or excoriation affecting exposed areas of skin, and bullous mastocytosis that typically presents as discrete pigmented papules and nodules with leathery induration and positive Darier sign [23, 24].

Based on the patient's history, physical examination, and skin biopsy with direct immunofluorescent result, this patient was diagnosed with infantile bullous pemphigoid. Bullous pemphigoid (BP) is an indolent autoimmune subepidermal blistering disorder characterized by large, tense blisters on erythematous or normal-appearing skin. This most frequently occurs in the elderly and is rarely seen in infants and children. There is no known racial or sexual predilection.

Infantile BP, which occurs in patients less than 1 year of age, predominantly affects acral skin and spares mucosal and genital surfaces [13, 14]. Pruritis is common [25] and may precede the appearance of the rash. Typical exam findings include tense bullae on erythematous or normal-appearing skin and filled with clear or hemorrhagic fluid [25]. The bullae may heal with milia formation but scarring generally does not occur. Nikolsky's sign is often absent [25]. Unlike in adults, the prognosis of infantile BP is favorable with almost all cases entering remission within 1 year of diagnosis [26].

Children over the age of 1 year who develop BP tend to have generalized disease with symmetrical, ungrouped blisters of variable size. The blisters are located primarily on flexural surfaces of the trunk and extremities. Older children with BP more commonly have mucosal involvement [14, 27]. There have been reports of vulvar adhesions and penile phimosis in older children with mucosal BP. Ocular involvement has a 25 % risk of blindness, whereas laryngeal disease has been known to cause airway compromise.

The pathogenesis of bullous pemphigoid in adults and children is similar. The skin lesions are due to the circulating and tissue-bound IgG autoantibodies directed against BP antigens 180 and 230 of the hemidesmosome adhesion complex in the basement membrane of the skin [13, 27].

BP has been associated with vaccination in infants. The theory is that the vaccine is believed to unmask a subclinical BP in genetically predisposed infants via a non-specific immune reactivation [13] while other authors speculate a cross-reaction between epidermal antigens and the immune response against viral or bacterial antigens [28]. However, review of the current pediatric literature revealed about 100 cases of childhood BP [29], only 18 of which occurred after vaccination [13]. Most of these patients did not have a recurrence of BP; only three of these patients had recurrence of disease on revaccination, all milder than the initial eruption [13]. Post-vaccination BP is therefore not considered a contraindication to repeat vaccination.

Histopathologic Findings

Skin biopsy taken from lesional skin demonstrates a subepidermal blister with eosinophils on H&E [27]. DIF of a perilesional skin may show linear deposition of IgG or C3 at the epidermal basement membrane zone [27]. Salt-split skin shows IgG deposition in the roof of the blister. There may also be circulating IgG against BP180 and BP230. Peripheral eosinophilia may also be seen.

Treatment

Infantile BP resolves rapidly upon initiation of therapy. Treatment of choice for infantile bullous pemphigoid is a topical or systemic steroid. For localized disease, topical steroids may be sufficient [30]. For extensive or severe disease when rapid resolution is needed, prednisone at 1–2 mg/kg/day may be started and tapered slowly with clearing [3, 30, 31]. A systemic antibiotic may be needed to treat secondarily infected lesions and erythromycin (50 mg/kg/day) with or without nicotinamide (40 mg/kg/day) have also been reported to be helpful for their anti-inflammatory effects [26, 30, 32]. Supplemental or alternative therapies for severe cases include dapsone (3–6 mg/kg/day, maximum dose 100 mg/day), sulfapyridine (2 mg/kg/day), and mycophenolate mofetil which serve as important steroid-sparing agents [26, 30]. For severe, recalcitrant disease, remission has been reported with IVIG or Rituximab (anti-CD20) [26, 30]. Extra-corporeal plasmapheresis and plasma exchange have also been found to be effective in the treatment of drug-resistant autoimmune diseases, although there are limited reports in the pediatric literature [26, 30]. As noted above, infantile BP is not a contraindication to subsequent vaccination. The family should be counselled that BP may recur after a subsequent vaccine as has been seen in a minority of cases. If steroids have been given, note that children receiving ≥2 mg/kg per day of prednisone, or ≥20 mg/day for 14 days or more, should not receive live virus vaccines for at least 1 month after discontinuation of corticosteroid therapy [33].

Conclusion

Bullous pemphigoid (BP) is an autoimmune subepidermal blistering condition that commonly affects the elderly but may occasionally affect infants and children. Clinically, the typical eruption is pruritic and is composed of urticarial plaques and large, tense ungrouped blisters of varying size on the flexural surfaces of the trunk and extremities. Histologically, there is a subepidermal blister with eosinophils on H&E and linear deposition of IgG or C3 at the epidermal basement membrane zone on DIF of perilesional skin. This condition responds well to topical or systemic steroids.

References

1. Sarkell B, Blaylock WK, Vernon H. Congenital neonatal herpes simplex infection. J Am Acad Dermatol. 1992;27(5):817–21.
2. Koch LH, Fisher RG, Chen C, Foster MM, Bass WT, William JV. Congenital herpes simplex virus infection: two unique cutaneous presentations associated with probable intrauterine transmission. J Am Acad Dermatol. 2009;60:312–5.
3. Paller A, Mancini A. Bullous disorders of childhood (Chapter 13). In: Paller AS, Mancini AJ, editors. Hurwitz clinical pediatric dermatology. 4th ed. Philadelphia: Elsevier; 2011.
4. Berk DR, Jazayeri L, Marinkovich MP, Sundram UN, Bruckner AL. Diagnosing epidermolysis bullosa type and subtype in infancy using immunofluorescence microscopy: the Stanford experience. Pediatr Dermatol. 2013;30(2):226–33.
5. Fine JD, Bruckner-Tuderman LB, Eady RA, Bauer EA, Bauer JW, Has C, et al. Inherited epidermolysis bullosa: updated recommendations on diagnosis and classification. J Am Acad Dermatol. 2014;70:1103–26.
6. Intong LRA, Murrell DF. How to take skin biopsies for epidermolysis bullosa. Dermatol Clin. 2010;28:197–200.
7. Takeichi T, Liu L, Fong K, Ozoemena L, McMillan JR, Salam A, Campbell P, Akiyama M, Mellerio JE, McLean WH, Simpson MA, McGrath JA. Whole-exome sequencing improves mutation detection in a diagnostic epidermolysis bullosa laboratory. Br J Dermatol. 2015;172(1):94–100.
8. Gonzalez ME. Evaluation and treatment of the newborn with epidermolysis bullosa. Semin Perinatol. 2013;37(1):32–9.
9. Eichenfield LF, Frieden IJ, editors. Neonatal and infant dermatology. 3rd ed. London: Elsevier Saunders; 2015.
10. Fortuna G, Marinkovich MP. Linear immunoglobulin A bullous dermatosis. Dermatol Clin. 2012;30:38–50.
11. Venning VA. Linear IgA disease: clinical presentation, diagnosis, and pathogenesis. Dermatol Clin. 2011;29:453–8.
12. Kneisel A, Hertl M. Autoimmune bullous skin diseases. Part 1: clinical manifestations. J German Soc Dermatol. 2011;10:844–57.
13. De la Fuente A, Hernández-Martin Á, et al. Postvaccination bullous pemphigoid in infancy: report of three new cases and literature review. Pediatr Dermatol. 2013;30(6):741–4.
14. Lynch M, Devaney D, et al. Bullae of the hands, feet, and perioral area in a 3-month-old infant. Pediatr Dermatol. 2013;30(1):135–6.
15. Prost-Squarcioni C, Caux F. Epidermolysis bullosa acquisita (Chapter 40). In: Murrell DF, editor. Blistering diseases: clinical features, pathogenesis, treatment. Sydney: Springer; 2015.
16. Léauté-Labrèze C, Lamireau T, Chawki D, Maleville J, Taïeb A. Diagnosis, classification, and management of erythema multiforme and Stevens–Johnson syndrome. Arch Dis Child. 2000;83:347–52.
17. Levin DL, Esterly NB, Herman JJ, Boxall LBH. The Sweet syndrome in children. J Pediatr. 1981;99(1):73–8.
18. Cooper SM, Powell J, Wojnarowska F. Linear IgA disease: successful treatment with erythromycin. Clin Exp Dermatol. 2002;27(8):677–9.
19. Siegfried EC, Sirawan S. Chronic bullous disease of childhood: successful treatment with dicloxacillin. J Am Acad Dermatol. 1998;35(5):797–800.

20. Mintz EM, Morel KD. Treatment of chronic bullous disease of childhood (Chapter 57). In: Murrell DF, editor. Blistering diseases: clinical features, pathogenesis, treatment. Sydney: Springer; 2015.
21. Edhegard K, Hall III R. Dapsone (Chapter 18). In: Wolverton SE, editor. Comprehensive dermatologic drug therapy. Philadelphia: Elsevier; 2013.
22. Ladhani S, Evans RW. Staphylococcal scalded skin syndrome. Arch Dis Child. 1998;78:85–8.
23. Howard R, Frieden IJ. Vesicles, pustules, bullae, erosions, and ulcerations (Chapter 10). In: Schachner LE, Frieden IJ, Esterly NB, editors. Neonatal and infant dermatology. Philadelphia: Elsevier; 2008.
24. Golitz LE, Weston WL, Lane AT. Bullous mastocytosis: diffuse cutaneous mastocytosis with extensive blisters mimicking scalded skin syndrome or erythema multiforme. Pediatr Dermatol. 1984;1(4):288–94.
25. Reis-Filho EG, Silva Tde A, et al. Bullous pemphigoid in a 3-month-old infant: case report and literature review of this dermatosis in childhood. An Bras Dermatol. 2013;88(6):961–5.
26. Weitz N, Mintz E, Morel K. Autoimmune bullous diseases of childhood (Chapter 5). In: Tom WL, editor. Severe skin diseases in children: beyond topical therapy. Berlin: Springer; 2014. p. 67–90.
27. Martinez-De Pablo MI, González-Enseñat MA, et al. Childhood bullous pemphigoid: clinical and immunological findings in a series of 4 cases. Arch Dermatol. 2007;143(2):215–20.
28. Amos BMD, Deng JS, et al. Bullous pemphigoid in infancy: case report and literature review. Pediatr Dermatol. 1998;15(2):108–11.
29. Marcus KA, Halbertsma FJ, van Steensel MA. A case of juvenile bullous pemphigoid—successful treatment with diaminodiphenylsulfone and prednisone. Pediatr Dermatol. 2009;26:55–8.
30. Simmons RN, Bruckner AL, Prok LD. Blisters in a 4-year-old: an unexpected diagnosis. Pediatr Dermatol. 2013;30(1):135–6.
31. Wolverton SE. Systemic corticosteroids (Chapter 12). In: Wolverton SE, editor. Comprehensive dermatologic drug therapy. Philadelphia: Elsevier; 2013.
32. Das D, Das A, Debbarman P. Childhood bullous pemphigoid. Indian Pediatr. 2013;50(12):1179.
33. Red Book®. 2015 report of the committee on infectious disease. 30th ed; 2015.

Chapter 13
Vasculitis

Marcia Hogeling

Abstract Childhood vasculitis includes a challenging group of conditions that often require multi-specialty care by dermatology, rheumatology, nephrology, cardiology, neurology, gastroenterology, and general pediatrics. Vasculitis in children may be from infection, autoimmune disorders, drug induced, related to malignancy, or idiopathic. A skin biopsy is essential for the diagnosis of many types of vasculitis. The most common type of childhood vasculitis is Henoch–Schönlein Purpura. This chapter discusses several types of pediatric vasculitis including Henoch–Schönlein Purpura, Polyarteritis nodosa, and Acute Hemorrhagic Edema of Infancy.

Keywords Vasculitis • Leukocytoclastic vasculitis • Panniculitis • Polyarteritis nodosa • Henoch–Schönlein Purpura • Acute hemorrhagic edema of infancy

Case 13.1

An 11-year-old previously healthy boy was admitted to hospital with fever and weakness. Over the past month, he had developed erythematous to purple tender plaques and nodules over his arms and legs, associated with joint pains and malaise. Several of these nodules healed leaving atrophic depressions on his skin. He denies abdominal pain, Raynaud phenomenon, or chest pain. He is not taking any medications.

Physical Exam (Fig. 13.1)

Vital signs: BP 110/80, HR 80, RR 20, temperature 102 °F.

M. Hogeling, MD (✉)
Division of Dermatology, University of California, Los Angeles,
52-121 CHS, 10833 Le Conte Ave, Los Angeles, CA 90095, USA
e-mail: hogelingm@yahoo.ca

© Springer International Publishing Switzerland 2016   221
M. Hogeling (ed.), *Case-Based Inpatient Pediatric Dermatology*,
DOI 10.1007/978-3-319-31569-0_13

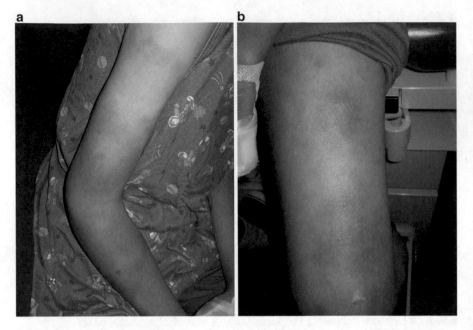

Fig. 13.1 (**a, b**) Erythematous to violaceous indurated tender plaques and nodules over the upper arms and legs. Background of livedo reticularis on the legs (**b**)

The child is generally ill appearing but not in acute distress. There are normal heart sounds, no heart murmurs, and chest is clear to auscultation. No masses are palpated on abdominal exam.

Laboratory Investigations

- White blood count 15 (4–10.5 K/μL)
- ESR 80 (0–20 mm/h)
- ANA negative
- Antiphospholipid antibodies negative
- Negative p-ANCA
- Negative c-ANCA
- Streptococcal titers negative

Questions

1. What is your differential diagnosis?
2. How would you treat this patient?

Answers

The differential diagnosis for erythematous nodules involving the arms and legs is broad and includes panniculitis such as erythema nodosum, vasculitis such as polyarteritis nodosa (PAN), Sweet syndrome, and infection such as disseminated bacterial and fungal infections. Vasculitis may be caused by infection, malignancy, or rheumatologic disorders [1].

An incisional skin biopsy of a new lesion was performed revealing fibrinoid necrosis and inflammation of small and medium-sized arteries in the deep dermis and subcutaneous fat. Biopsy for direct immunofluorescence showed deposition of IgM and C3, consistent with a diagnosis of PAN.

There are several types of PAN including PAN with systemic organ involvement (PAN) and benign cutaneous polyarteritis nodosa (BPAN). PAN is a necrotizing vasculitis of small and medium-sized arteries that is quite uncommon in children and is classified as to whether it is limited to cutaneous involvement versus whether there is systemic involvement. Prognosis is correlated with the degree of additional organ involvement, which may include joints, muscles, kidneys, heart, GI tract, and rarely cerebral infarcts. Cutaneous features may include subcutaneous nodules, palpable purpura, livedoracemosa, retiform purpura, ulcerations, and digital infarcts. Nodules may heal, leaving atrophic plaques. Further workup of this child revealed lack of internal organ involvement, consistent with the subtype of BPAN. BPAN is limited to the skin and is the most common type of PAN in children. Patients may have mild systemic symptoms such as fever, myalgias, and arthralgias. Cutaneous PAN may be associated with streptococcal infections. Although BPAN may have a chronic, relapsing course, it has a better prognosis than systemic PAN. A significant complication of BPAN is digital or extremity necrosis [2].

Treatment of BPAN is with high-dose systemic corticosteroids initially, (such as 1 mg/kg/day of prednisone) that is gradually tapered over months. In mild cases, NSAIDS may be used, but typically systemic corticosteroids are required. Steroid sparing immunosuppressive drugs such as cyclophosphamide and mycophenolate mofetil may be used second line [3]. There are case reports of treatment with colchicine, dapsone, cyclophosphamide, methotrexate, anti-TNF agents, IVIG, and mycophenolate mofetil [4–7]. There is controversy over whether cutaneous PAN may be induced by streptococcal infection. Patients with proven streptococcal infections are frequently treated with long-term penicillin prophylaxis; however, evidence for this is unclear [8]. For systemic disease, treatment in conjunction with a Pediatric Rheumatologist is critical.

Case 13.2

A 12-year-old Hispanic female presented with a 10-day history of a purplish rash that began on her left leg and spread to her abdomen and upper extremities. She had associated knee pain, myalgia, abdominal pain, nausea, and non-bloody, non-bilious emesis. Her past medical history was significant for MRSA abscesses, the most recent of which was treated with trimethoprim-sulfamethoxazole; she finished treatment 5 days before the onset of this rash. Family history was significant for her aunt who died of systemic lupus.

Physical Exam (Fig. 13.2)

Physical exam showed erythematous macules and purpuric papules with central vesiculation extending up her thighs, lower abdomen, and distal upper extremities, associated with edema of her lower extremities and significant pain to palpation. There were tense bullae on her distal lower extremities.

Laboratory Investigations

- CBC normal
- ANA-negative
- dsDNA-negative
- Liver enzymes-normal
- Urinalysis-normal

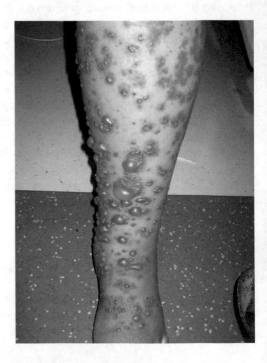

Fig. 13.2 Tense bullae superimposed over purpura on the lower extremities

Questions

1. What is the diagnosis?
2. How would you treat this patient?
3. What is a potential long-term complication to be aware of with this condition?

Answers

The skin biopsy (Fig. 13.3) shows an intense inflammatory infiltrate of neutrophils around blood vessels within the dermis. These blood vessels showed swollen endothelium and narrowing of the vessel lumina. Direct immunofluorescence revealed granular IgA, C3, fibrin, and weak IgM deposits in blood vessels in the papillary dermis consistent with Henoch–Schönlein Purpura (HSP). HSP is a small vessel, leukocytoclastic vasculitis caused by immune complex deposition. Direct immunofluorescence is positive for granular deposits of IgA, which help distinguish it from other types of leukocytoclastic vasculitis. The differential diagnosis includes other types of leukocytoclastic vasculitis and disseminated bacterial and viral infections with petechiae and purpura, such as meningococcemia. For this patient, with the history of prior infection and antibiotic use, we considered vasculitis caused by infection, or hypersensitivity from drugs. Given the family history of autoimmune disease, autoimmune causes such as systemic lupus erythematosus were also investigated, and found to be negative.

This patient has bullae on the lower extremities, superimposed over the purpura, a clinical variant of *bullous* Henoch–Schönlein Purpura. Bullous HSP is more common in adults than children.

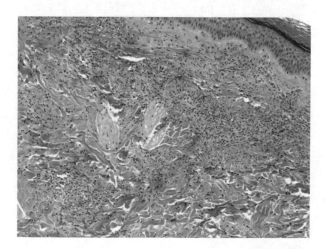

Fig. 13.3 Perivascular inflammatory infiltrate of neutrophils around blood vessels within the dermis with leukocytoclasis associated with endothelial swelling and narrowing of the vessel lumina. (Courtesy Daphne DeMello, MD)

HSP is the most common type of vasculitis seen in children. It typically affects younger children between the ages of 4 and 6, with an incidence of 13 per 100,000 [9]. A classic triad includes abdominal pain, arthralgias, and a purpuric eruption. Renal involvement is less common.

Treatment for HSP is generally supportive care. Children with mild skin involvement do not need treatment. Systemic steroids may be utilized for severe abdominal pain and may reduce the chance of persistent renal involvement. Bullous lesions are another indication for systemic corticosteroids although this is somewhat controversial [10, 11]. This patient was treated with prednisone, with improvement in skin pain and decreased bullae within several days.

A potential long-term complication is renal disease which develops within 6 months of the purpura in the majority of patients; therefore, serial monitoring of urinalysis is indicated. Routine blood pressure and urinalysis are recommended for 6 months [1, 9].

Case 13.3

A 6-month-old previously healthy boy presents to the hospital with a fever, swelling of the face and hands, and skin rash affecting the face, ears, and extremities. The rash has been present for 2 days, starting as small red-purple spots that are enlarging. He is irritable and not feeding well. He has not been taking any medications. The past week he has had rhinorrhea and some diarrhea.

Physical Exam (Fig. 13.4)

He is generally well appearing. The facial edema seems to be painful but non-pitting.

Laboratory Investigations

- Leukocytosis
- Elevated ESR
- Urinalysis normal

Question

1. What is the diagnosis?

Fig. 13.4 Multiple circular red-purple ecchymotic papules and plaques, coalescing into polycyclic and annular plaques, over the face, ears, arms, and legs

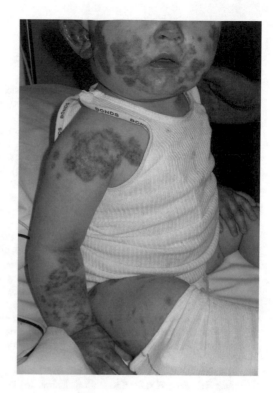

Answers

The correct diagnosis is acute hemorrhagic edema of infancy (AHEI). AHEI is a benign vasculitis (leukocytoclastic vasculitis) affecting young children, typically between 4 months and 2 years of age, that is slightly more common in males [12, 13]. The etiology is unclear, but involves immune complex deposition. It is thought to be similar to HSP; however, it can be differentiated by the circular nature of the purpura, as well as the location favoring the face and arms, rather than legs and buttocks as seen in HSP. Lesions may be described as "cockade" or targetoid consisting of annular lesions with darker centers. Skin biopsy findings do not always show IgA deposition, (as opposed to HSP) leading to the controversy of whether this condition is separate from HSP, or an infantile variant [13].

The differential diagnosis includes infection such as meningococcemia, causes of ecchymosis such as child abuse, Kawasaki disease, and HSP.

There is often a preceding history of upper respiratory infection, or GI symptoms such as diarrhea or vomiting. While the rash is dramatic, the infants often appear otherwise well. There is often facial swelling, and ecchymotic purpura of the face and extremities.

Given the self-limited nature of the disease, with no long-term effects on renal function, treatment is unnecessary.

The condition has a good prognosis and the skin eruption generally resolves within 1–3 weeks [1].

References

1. Ting TV. Diagnosis and management of cutaneous vasculitis in children. Pediatr Clin North Am. 2014;61(2):321–46.
2. Williams VL, Guirola R, Flemming K, et al. Distal extremity necrosis as a manifestation of cutaneous polyarteritis nodosa; case report and review of the acute management of a pediatric patient. Pediatr Dermatol. 2012;29(4):473–8.
3. Merlin E, Mouy R, Pereira B, Mouthon L, et al. Long term outcome of children with pediatric onset cutaneous and visceral polyarteritis nodosa. Joint Bone Spine. 2015;10(3):e0120981.
4. Zoshima T, Matsumura M, Suzuki Y, et al. A case of refractory cutaneous polyarteritis nodosa in a patient with hepatitis B carrier status successfully treated with tumor necrosis factor alpha blockade. Mod Rheumatol. 2013;23(5):1029–33.
5. Schartz NE, Alaoui S, Vignon-Pennamen MD, et al. Successful treatment in two cases of steroid-dependent cutaneous polyarteritis nodosa with low-dose methotrexate. Dermatology. 2001;203(4):336–8.
6. Lobo I, Ferreira M, Silva E, et al. Cutaneous polyarteritis nodosa treated with intravenous immunoglobulins. J Eur Acad Dermatol Venereol. 2008;22(7):880–2.
7. Kluger N, Guillot B, Bessis D. Ulcerative cutaneous polyarteritis nodosa treated with mycophenolate mofetil and pentoxifylline. J Dermatolog Treat. 2011;22(3):175–7.
8. Till SH, Amos RS. Long-term follow-up of juvenile-onset cutaneous polyarteritis nodosa associated with streptococcal infection. Br J Rheumatol. 1997;36(8):909–11.
9. Stewart M, Savage JM, Bell B, McCord B. Long term renal prognosis of Henoch-Schonlein purpura in an unselected childhood population. Eur J Pediatr. 1988;147:113–5.
10. den Boer SL, Pasmans SG, Wulffraat NM, Ramakers-Van Woerden NL, Bousema MT. Bullous lesions in Henoch Schönlein Purpura as indication to start systemic prednisone. Acta Paediatr. 2010;99(5):781–3. doi:10.1111/j.1651-2227.2009.01650.x. Epub 2009 Jan 5.
11. Chan KH, Tang WY, Lo KK. Bullous lesions in Henoch-Schönlein purpura. Pediatr Dermatol. 2007;24(3):325–6.
12. Savino F, Lupica MM, Tarasco V, et al. Acute hemorrhagic edema of infancy: a troubling cutaneous presentation with a self limiting course. Pediatr Dermatol. 2013;30(6):3149–52.
13. Fiore E, Rizzi M, Ragazzi M, et al. Acute hemorrhagic edema of young children (cockade purpura and edema); a case series and systematic review. J Am Acad Dermatol. 2008;59(4):684–95.

Chapter 14
Skin Signs of Systemic Diseases

Adam Bartlett, Pamela Palasanthiran, Marcia Hogeling, and Orli Wargon

Abstract This chapter discusses examples of neutrophilic dermatoses and panniculitides, which represent a spectrum of non-infectious inflammatory conditions of the epidermis, dermis, and subcutaneous tissue. They can be associated with systemic diseases, including malignancies, and autoimmune and autoinflammatory disorders. Histopathological examination of the lesions is integral to the diagnosis of these cutaneous or subcutaneous inflammatory conditions. Treatment includes management of the associated systemic disease, in conjunction with a range of anti-inflammatory and immune-modulatory therapies.

Keywords Neutrophilic dermatosis • Sweet's syndrome • Pyoderma gangrenosum • Panniculitis • Cutaneous findings of systemic disease

Case 14.1

History

A 13-year-old girl diagnosed with acute myeloid leukemia (AML) 2 weeks prior, currently admitted for induction chemotherapy, developed multiple well-demarcated, erythematous and tender plaques on her left flank. She had been febrile for the previous

A. Bartlett, BSc, MBBS, MPHTM (✉) • P. Palasanthiran, MBBS, MD, FRACP
Department of Immunology and Infectious Diseases, Sydney Children's Hospital,
High Street, Randwick, NSW 2031, Australia
e-mail: adam.bartlett@health.nsw.gov.au; pamela.palasanthiran@health.nsw.gov.au

M. Hogeling, MD
Division of Dermatology, University of California, Los Angeles,
52-121 CHS, 10833 Le Conte Ave, Los Angeles, CA 90095, USA
e-mail: hogelingm@yahoo.ca

O. Wargon, MBBS (Hons1), MClin, Ed, FACD
Department Paediatric Dermatology, Sydney Children's Hospital,
High Street, Randwick, NSW 2031, Australia
e-mail: orli.wargon@health.nsw.gov.au

© Springer International Publishing Switzerland 2016
M. Hogeling (ed.), *Case-Based Inpatient Pediatric Dermatology*,
DOI 10.1007/978-3-319-31569-0_14

229

3 days without evidence of sepsis. Her medications at the time included ondansetron, metoclopramide, gentamicin, piperacillin–tazobactam, trimethoprim–sulfamethoxazole, and liposomal amphotericin. She had completed a 10-day cycle of chemotherapy (cytarabine, daunorubicin, and etoposide) the day before. No granulocyte-colony stimulating factor (G-CSF) was given. Within 24 h more lesions of a similar nature had developed on her left thigh, left hip, and back.

Physical Examination (Fig. 14.1)

On examination, there were multiple tender, warm, erythematous plaques (six in total) measuring 2×2 cm on her left flank, left thigh, left hip, and back. The lesions were slightly raised and indurated, but non-fluctuant. She was febrile and had rigors. There was no evidence of mucosal lesions or visceromegaly.

Investigations

- Hb 105 g/L (115–165 g/L)
- WCC 2.30×10^9 L^{-1} (3.50–11.00×10^9 L^{-1})

Fig. 14.1 Photo of bilateral infra-orbital lesions which developed 8 days after original skin lesions

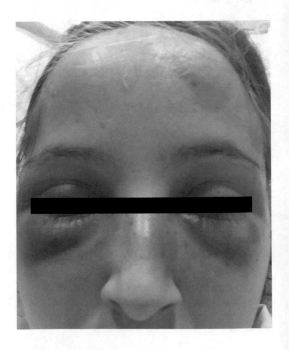

- Platelets 37×10^9 L^{-1} (150–450×10^9 L^{-1})
- Neutrophils 1.9×10^9 L^{-1} (1.7–7.0×10^9 L^{-1})
- Lymphocytes 0.3×10^9 L^{-1} (1.5–4.0×10^9 L^{-1})
- Eosinophils 0.00×10^9 L^{-1} (0.04–0.44×10^9 L^{-1})

Questions

1. What would you include in your differential diagnoses?
2. What further investigations would you order?
3. What treatment options would you consider?

Patient Progress

The patient's antibiotic regimen was changed to meropenem and vancomycin; the liposomal amphotericin was increased from prophylactic to treatment doses; and her prophylactic trimethoprim–sulfamethoxazole was continued. Serial blood cultures remained negative, and an autoimmune screen (ANA and eNA) was unremarkable. A CT of her chest, abdomen, and pelvis demonstrated consolidation and ground glass opacification in the upper lobe of the right lung, suggestive of fungal infection.

A biopsy of one of the skin lesions on her flank demonstrated epidermal spongiosis, hyperkeratosis, and acanthosis, with a light neutrophilic infiltrate. Intraepidermal and subcorneal pustules containing neutrophils, as well as an interstitial and perivascular mixed inflammatory (neutrophilic and lymphocytic) infiltrate in the superficial dermis, were also evident. These features are consistent with a spongiotic and pustular dermatitis, suggestive of an infection or neutrophilic dermatosis. Fungal spores (with a morphological appearance consistent with *Malassezia furfur*) were seen in the most superficial layers of the stratum corneum, with no extension into the epidermis or dermis. No other bacterial, fungal, or acid-fast organisms were identified on histopathology, microscopy, or culture.

Over the subsequent 7 days the lesions on her flank, hip, thigh, and back settled. On day 8 following the original skin lesion, bilateral infraorbital erythema, swelling, and tenderness developed, which evolved into a purpuric appearance, then faded over several days (Fig. 14.1). A CT of her sinuses did not demonstrate any evidence of sinusitis and her eyesight was not impacted. Her fevers settled after 16 days, at which time the antibiotics (meropenem and vancomycin) were ceased, and she was commenced on voriconazole for ongoing treatment of an invasive fungal infection.

Answer

The neutrophilic dermatoses are a group of noninfectious skin conditions characterized by cutaneous lesions with intense sterile neutrophilic inflammation [1, 2]. In this case, the clinicopathologic diagnosis of acute febrile neutrophilic dermatosis, or Sweet's syndrome, was made. Patients can present with a range of cutaneous manifestations, which generally involve tender, well-demarcated, erythematous lesions (e.g., papules, plaques, pustules, bullae, nodules) that may become hemorrhagic but usually resolve without scarring [3]. Fever often precedes the skin lesions, while conjunctivitis and episcleritis can also occur [3, 4]. Rarely, post-inflammatory cutis laxa-like slack skin with arterial laxity can follow Sweet's syndrome. Differential diagnoses include infection (viral, bacterial, fungal, mycobacterial) and vasculitis.

The definitive diagnosis of Sweet's syndrome requires two major and at least two minor criteria (Table 14.1) [3, 4]. Central to diagnosis is biopsy and histopathological examination of a skin lesion demonstrating an intense infiltrate of polymorphonuclear leukocytes localizing to the epidermis, dermis, or hypodermis [5]. In pancytopenic patients receiving chemotherapy, such as in this case, less inflammatory cells may be present. The localization of cutaneous neutrophilic inflammation in association with other systemic and extra-cutaneous manifestations assists in specifying a particular neutrophilic dermatosis. However, overlap forms and concurrent or successive neutrophilic dermatoses do occur [3, 6].

Neutrophilic dermatoses are often idiopathic but may be associated with many systemic disorders including myeloproliferative disorders, monoclonal gammopathies, inflammatory bowel disease, and auto-immune and auto-inflammatory disorders [1, 3, 7]. AML is the most common malignancy associated with Sweet's syndrome [8]. These secondary causes need to be considered during the diagnostic process, as they have significant implications for long-term management and prognosis. Several medications (e.g., trimethoprim–sulfamethoxazole, granulocyte colony-stimulating factor, all-trans retinoic acid) have been reported with cases of Sweet's syndrome; however these are usually administered in association with underlying malignancy or inflammatory disorders [3, 9, 10].

Table 14.1 Diagnostic criteria for Sweet's syndrome[a]

Major criteria	Minor criteria
• Acute onset of erythematous or violaceous plaques or nodules	• Preceding fever or infection
• Predominantly neutrophilic dermal infiltration without leukocytoclastic vasculitis	• Accompanying fever, arthralgia, conjunctivitis, or underlying malignancy
	• Responds to systemic corticosteroids, but not antibiotics
	• Raised white cell count
	• Raised erythrocyte sedimentation rate

[a]Adapted from Dabade and Davis [9]

A range of treatment options exist for the various neutrophilic dermatoses, and include systemic, topical, and intralesional therapies. The main principal of treatment is to manage the inflammatory process through anti-inflammatory, immuno-suppressive, and immunomodulatory agents [3, 6, 9]. Systemic corticosteroids are usually effective; however with recurrences other agents such as potassium iodide, colchicine, and dapsone have been used [6, 9]. Treatment should be tailored to the individual, taking into account the associated systemic disorder and systemic involvement during the episode. In some patients with Sweet's syndrome the lesions may spontaneously resolve without therapeutic intervention [8]. Recurrences may occur, particularly in malignancy-associated Sweet's syndrome, where the lesions represent a paraneoplastic phenomenon and may signify a malignancy relapse [8].

Case 14.2

History

A 17-year-old boy diagnosed with acute lymphoblastic leukemia (ALL) 13 months prior presents to the Emergency Department with a tender, non-fluctuant, slightly raised, erythematous lesion, measuring 2 cm in diameter on his left upper arm (Fig. 14.2). Management of his ALL had been complicated by asparaginase-induced

Fig. 14.2 Erythematous plaque on upper left arm

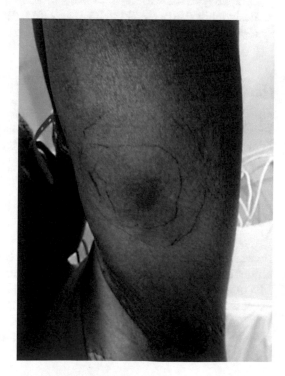

pancreatitis, a pulmonary invasive fungal infection, extensive herpes simplex sto-matitis, and anaphylaxis to liposomal amphotericin. His medications at the time included voriconazole, acyclovir, co-trimoxazole, thioguanine, esomeprazole, and dexamethasone (recently weaned). He had received cytarabine, cyclophosphamide, and intrathecal methotrexate as part of his chemotherapy protocol 4 days earlier.

Physical Examination

On presentation the patient was afebrile and reported abdominal pain. Aside from the skin lesion on his left upper arm, the remainder of his examination was unremarkable.

Investigations

- Hb 115 g/L (130–180 g/L)
- WCC 0.39×10^9 L^{-1} (3.50–11.00×10^9 L^{-1})
- Platelets 75×10^9 L^{-1} (150–450×10^9 L^{-1})
- Neutrophils 0.1×10^9 L^{-1} (1.7–7.0×10^9 L^{-1})
- Lymphocytes 0.2×10^9 L^{-1} (1.5–4.0×10^9 L^{-1})
- Eosinophils 0.00×10^9 L^{-1} (0.04–0.44×10^9 L^{-1})
- C-reactive protein 212 mg/L (<3 mg/L)

Questions

1. What would you include in your differential diagnoses?
2. What further investigations would you order?
3. What treatment options would you consider?

Patient Progress

He was admitted to hospital and commenced on broad spectrum antibiotics (piper-acillin–tazobactam and gentamicin) and continued his regular medications. Within 24 h of his admission, he developed fevers and the lesion became more painful and increased in size. Similar lesions developed on his scalp, both arms and legs, and back (total of nine lesions). His antibacterial and antifungal cover was broadened with meropenem, vancomycin, co-trimoxazole, and liposomal amphotericin (via a desensitization protocol due to his previous anaphylactic reaction). He required opioid analgesia and was commenced on G-CSF.

Ultrasound of the original lesion on his left upper arm demonstrated diffuse edema in the subcutaneous fat plane, without a collection or mass. His lipase and amylase were not elevated, serial blood cultures negative, and an autoimmune screen (ANA, eNA, dsDNA, ANCA, C3, C4) was unremarkable. Biopsies were taken from lesions on the right and left upper arm. They demonstrated identical features of deep dermal and subcutaneous inflammation with a mixed lymphocytic and neutrophilic infiltrate, consistent with septal panniculitis. *Micrococcus luteus* was identified on culture, which was considered to be non-pathogenic. No other bacterial, fungal, or acid-fast organisms were identified on histopathology, microscopy, or culture. The lesions and fevers settled by day 9 of his admission and he was discharged 2 days later with slight residual erythema at the site of the lesions.

Answer

Panniculitis is a condition that is characterized by inflammation of the subcutaneous adipose tissue [11]. It can occur as a primary phenomenon, a local reaction, secondary to medications, or as part of a systemic disorder (Table 14.2) [12–15]. Despite the diverse nature of associated etiologies, patients present in a similar fashion with painful and tender erythematous nodules or plaques that are usually located on the lower limbs, but can occur anywhere [12]. Patients may have other nonspecific symptoms such as fever and lethargy, as well as more specific features indicative of an associated underlying condition. Differential diagnoses include infection and vasculitis (polyarteritis nodosa).

Table 14.2 Causes of panniculitis

Erythema nodosum (most common)	Connective tissue disease
Beta-hemolytic streptococcus	Systemic lupus erythematosus
Mycoplasma	Dermatomyositis
Epstein–Barr virus	Polyarteritis nodosa
Sarcoidosis	**Enzymatic**
Drugs: oral contraceptives, sulphonamides, penicillin, cephalosporins, macrolides	Pancreatitis
Infections	α_1-Antitrypsin deficiency
Bacterial	**Physical**
Fungal	Trauma
Mycobacterial	Cold
Malignancy	**Post-steroids**
Leukemia	**Subcutaneous fat necrosis of the newborn**
Lymphoma (T-cell)	

Biopsy and histopathological examination of the lesion is necessary for the definitive diagnosis of panniculitis [15]. Classification systems, based on the location of inflammation (septal, lobular, or mixed) and other associated features (e.g., vasculitis, necrosis, cellular infiltrate), assist in guiding the clinician to an underlying etiology, however significant overlap exists [14–18]. Given the homogenous clinical presentation of panniculitis and the heterogeneity of associated etiologies, an understanding of the histopathology is important in determining a cause, and guiding further investigations and management. Other investigations will be guided by clinical suspicion and suggestive histopathological findings, but may include microbiological investigations, lipase, α_1-antitrypsin, autoimmune antibodies, and investigations for autoinflammatory disorders.

Treatment of panniculitis is generally supportive in nature in addition to directed therapy aimed at the underlying cause. Anti-inflammatory agents (nonsteroidal and corticosteroids) are used in select cases [12]. Some lesions will tend to resolve over 4–6 weeks without residual scar formation [11], especially post-steroid panniculitis, which develops 2–4 weeks after suddenly stopping systemic corticosteroids. Significant lipoatrophy can occur with lobular panniculitis, such as seen with systemic lupus erythematosus, deep morphoea, and juvenile dermatomyositis [18]. Lipoatrophy is also a feature of associated autoinflammatory disorders such as H-syndrome (SLC29A3 mutation) and chronic atypical neutrophilic dermatosis with lipodystrophy and elevated temperature (CANDLE) syndrome [19]. Deep necrotic ulceration is a feature of α_1-antitrypsin deficiency panniculitis seen mainly in homozygotes [15]. Pancreatic panniculitis tends to ulcerate and heal with atrophic scars [15].

Case 14.3

History

A 12-year-old unvaccinated girl presents to the Emergency Department with a 3-day history of a vesiculo-pustular eruption involving the trunk, extremities, scalp, and face.

She has a past medical history significant for MRSA infection and inflammatory bowel disease. She is taking prednisone for Crohn's disease and her dose is slowly being tapered. A purulent lesion on her right arm was incised and drained in the emergency room. It is now enlarging, sloughing, and extremely painful. Due to concerns for acute bacterial or viral infection in an immunocompromised patient, she was admitted to hospital and started on broad spectrum IV antibiotics, and IV acyclovir.

Physical Examination (Figs. 14.3 and 14.4)

Fig. 14.3 Vesicles, bullae, and pustules distributed over the arms and legs

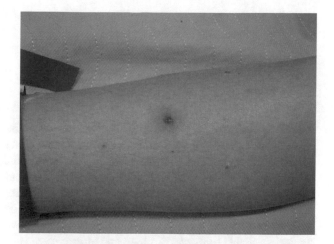

Fig. 14.4 Necrotic plaque, studded with peripheral pustules, central ulcer with undermined border, and surrounding rim of inflammation, corresponding to the site of previous incision and drainage

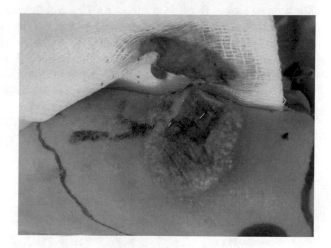

Investigations

- White blood cell count 17.1 (4.0–10.5 K/μL)
- Neutrophils 13.8 (1.0–8.9 K/μL)
- CRP 16.8 (<0.9 mg/dL)
- Varicella PCR negative
- Viral wound culture negative
- Bacterial culture from arm negative

Questions

1. What additional investigations would you perform?
2. What is the diagnosis?

3. Why did the ulcer on the wrist (Fig. 14.4) worsen?
4. What treatment do you recommend?

Discussion

Additional investigations to help with diagnosis would be to perform a skin biopsy of an active skin lesion with sufficient depth (to subcutaneous fat) and sufficient tissue for special stains and culture (bacterial, mycobacterial, fungal and viral). Other investigations depending on the clinical presentation could include gastrointestinal workup with colonoscopy and liver function tests, CBC, serology for ANA, antiphospholipid antibodies, ANCA antibodies, and VDRL. A skin biopsy was performed from a new pustule, revealing a dense neutrophilic infiltrate extending to the base of the lesion. Stains for bacteria, fungi, and viruses were negative. There was no vasculitis seen on biopsy (Figs. 14.5 and 14.6). Tissue cultures showed no growth.

The clinical findings, together with the biopsy findings, are consistent with a diagnosis of pyoderma gangrenosum (PG), which is a neutrophilic dermatosis. Neutrophilic skin infiltrations usually indicate infection, but neutrophilic dermatoses are disorders without primary skin infection. The differential diagnosis includes bullous Sweet's syndrome (another neutrophilic dermatosis that can mimic bullous PG), systemic vasculitis such as periarteritis nodosa, mycobacterial and atypical mycobacterial infections, syphilis, brown recluse spider bites, and systemic mycoses such as blastomycosis, sporotrichosis, coccidioidomycosis, and cryptococcosis.

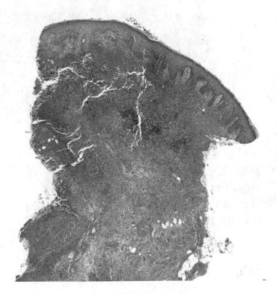

Fig. 14.5 Low power microscopic view showing biopsy from edge of ulcer with dense cellular infiltrate extending to the base of the lesion

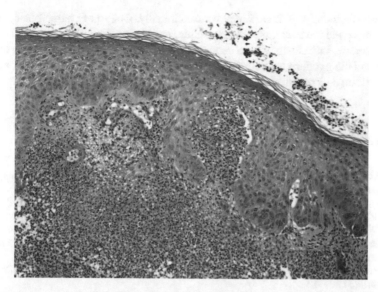

Fig. 14.6 Higher power microscopic view showing dense neutrophilic infiltrate without vasculitis

The classic morphology of pyoderma gangrenosum is an ulcer. It can present with a single lesion or multiple lesions. The initial lesion usually begins as a tender papulopustule that undergoes necrosis and ulcerates. It then heals with scarring which may be cribriform. It is more common in adults with only 4 % of cases presenting in children [20]. Clinical variants include bullous, pustular, superficial, and granulomatous/vegetative morphologies. Painful cutaneous lesions may occur anywhere on the body. Vesiculobullous pyoderma gangrenosum overlaps with superficial bullous Sweet's syndrome [7].

The ulcer on the wrist worsened due to a phenomenon called *pathergy*. Pathergy is the development of lesions at sites of minor trauma, which may occur in up to 20 % of cases. Pathergy is more common in childhood disease than in adult PG [20]. Some clinicians are concerned about performing biopsies in children with PG due to inducing pathergy, however biopsy is still recommended, to rule out other conditions. Biopsy from the edge of the ulcer can help rule out vasculitis. Biopsy from the ulcer itself can be submitted for culture—and in this case there was a high level of concern about infection from the primary care team, which was ruled out by the biopsy.

Pyoderma gangrenosum usually develops in conjunction with systemic disease, most commonly inflammatory bowel disease, but can also be seen in patients with arthritis, hematologic malignancies (leukemia), immunodeficiencies and autoinflammatory diseases such as pyogenic arthritis pyoderma gangrenosum, and acne (PAPA) syndrome [7].

Treatment of pyoderma gangrenosum includes systemic corticosteroids, and steroid sparing immunosuppressive drugs such as cyclosporine and TNF alpha inhibitors. A randomized trial in adults comparing prednisone and cyclosporine found that they were both about equally effective [21]. For a single PG lesion, topical or intralesional steroids or topical calcineurin inhibitors may be used initially. Due to her numerous cutaneous lesions, this patient was continued on systemic steroids, and switched to pulsed IV methylprednisolone. Infliximab was subsequently added to treat both the underlying Crohn's disease and the pyoderma gangrenosum [22, 23]. She had complete healing of her skin lesions within 2–3 months of therapy and was tapered off of systemic steroids.

References

1. Prat L, Bouaziz JD, Wallach D, Vignon-Pennamen MD, Bagot M. Neutrophilic dermatoses as systemic diseases. Clin Dermatol. 2014;32(3):376–88.
2. Saavedra AP, Kovacs SC, Moschella SL. Neutrophilic dermatoses. Clin Dermatol. 2006;24(6):470–81.
3. Berk D, Bayliss SJ. Neutrophilic dermatoses in children. Pediatr Dermatol. 2008;25(5):509–19.
4. Su WP, Liu HN. Diagnostic criteria for Sweet's syndrome. Cutis. 1986;37(3):167–74.
5. Sutra-Loubet C, Carlotti A, Guillemette J, Wallach D. Neutrophilic panniculitis. J Am Acad Dermatol. 2004;50(2):280–5.
6. Cohen PR. Neutrophilic dermatoses: a review of current treatment options. Am J Clin Dermatol. 2009;10(5):301–12.
7. Webb K, Hlela C, Jordaan HF, Suliman S, Scriba T, Lipsker D, Scott C. A review and proposed approach to the neutrophilic dermatoses of childhood. Pediatr Dermatol. 2015;32(4):437–46.
8. Cohen PR. Sweet's syndrome—a comprehensive review of an acute febrile neutrophilic dermatosis. Orphanet J Rare Dis. 2007;2:34.
9. Dabade TS, Davis MDP. Diagnosis and treatment of the neutrophilic dermatoses (pyoderma gangrenosum, Sweet's syndrome). Dermatol Ther. 2011;24(2):273–84.
10. Fazili TJ, Duncan D, Wanji L. Sweet's syndrome. Am J Med. 2010;123(8):694–6.
11. Moraes AJP, Soares PMF, Zapata AL, Lotito APN, Sallum AME, Silva CAA. Panniculitis in childhood and adolescence. Pediatr Int. 2006;48(1):48–53.
12. Torrelo A, Hernandez A. Panniculitis in children. Dermatol Clin. 2008;26(4):491–500.
13. Delgado-Jimenez Y, Fraga J, Garcia-Diez A. Infective panniculitis. Dermatol Clin. 2008;26(4):471–80.
14. Chan MP. Neutrophilic panniculitis: algorithmic approach to a heterogeneous group of disorders. Arch Pathol Lab Med. 2014;138(10):1337–43.
15. Polcari IC, Stein SL. Panniculitis in childhood. Dermatol Ther. 2010;23(4):356–67.
16. Diaz Cascajo C, Borghi S, Weyers W. Panniculitis: definition of terms and diagnostic strategy. Am J Dermatopathol. 2000;22(6):530–49.
17. Requena L, Yus ES. Panniculitis. Part I. Mostly septal panniculitis. J Am Acad Dermatol. 2001;45(2):163–83.
18. Requena LR, Yus ES. Panniculitis. Part II. Mostly lobular panniculitis. J Am Acad Dermatol. 2001;45(3):325–61.
19. Torrelo A, Patel S, Colmenero I, Gurbindo D, Lendinez F, Hernandez A, et al. Chronic atypical neutrophilic dermatosis with lipodystrophy and elevated temperature (CANDLE) syndrome. J Am Acad Dermatol. 2010;62(3):489–95.
20. Powell FC, Su WPD, Perry HO. Pyoderma gangrenosum: classification and management. J Am Acad Dermtol. 1996;34:395–409.
21. Ormerod AD, Thomas KS, Craig FE, et al. Comparison of the two most commonly used treatments for pyoderma gangrenosum: results of the STOP GAP randomised controlled trial. BMJ. 2015;350:h2958. doi:10.1136/bmj.h2958.
22. Nozawa T, Hara R, Kinoshita J, et al. Infliximab for a girl with refractory pyoderma gangrenosum. Nihon Rinsho Meneki Gakkai Kaishi. 2008;31:454–9.
23. Kaur MR, Lewis HM. Severe recalcitrant pyoderma gangrenosum treated with infliximab. Br J Dermatol. 2005;153:689–91.

Index

© Springer International Publishing Switzerland 2016
M. Hogeling (ed.), *Case-Based Inpatient Pediatric Dermatology*,
DOI 10.1007/978-3-319-31569-0

Printed in the United States
By Bookmasters